YOUR BEST
BRAIN
EVER

YOUR BEST
BRAIN
EVER

A COMPLETE GUIDE & WORKOUT

MICHAEL S. SWEENEY
Including "Brain Boosters" by Cynthia R. Green, Ph.D.

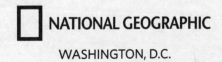

NATIONAL GEOGRAPHIC

WASHINGTON, D.C.

Published by the National Geographic Society
1145 17th Street N.W., Washington, D.C. 20036

All art by Jameson Simpson

Library of Congress Cataloging-in-Publication Data

Sweeney, Michael S.
  Your best brain ever : a complete guide and workout / Michael S. Sweeney, including "Brain Boosters" by Cynthia R. Green, Ph.D.
      p. cm.
  Includes bibliographical references and index.
  ISBN 978-1-4262-1170-6 (pbk.)
  1. Brain--Diseases--Prevention--Popular works. 2. Brain--Aging--Prevention--Popular works. 3. Intellect--Problems, exercises, etc. 4. Baby boom generation--Life skills guides. I. Green, Cynthia R. II. Title.
  RC386.2.S79 2013
  616.805--dc23
                                    2013028052

The National Geographic Society is one of the world's largest nonprofit scientific and educational organizations. Founded in 1888 to "increase and diffuse geographic knowledge," the Society's mission is to inspire people to care about the planet. It reaches more than 400 million people worldwide each month through its official journal, National Geographic, and other magazines; National Geographic Channel; television documentaries; music; radio; films; books; DVDs; maps; exhibitions; live events; school publishing programs; interactive media; and merchandise. National Geographic has funded more than 10,000 scientific research, conservation and exploration projects and supports an education program promoting geographic literacy.

For more information, visit www.nationalgeographic.com.

National Geographic Society
1145 17th Street N.W.
Washington, D.C. 20036-4688 U.S.A.

For information about special discounts for bulk purchases, please contact National Geographic Books Special Sales: ngspecsales@ngs.org

For rights or permissions inquiries, please contact National Geographic Books Subsidiary Rights: ngbookrights@ngs.org

Interior design: Melissa Farris/Katie Olsen

Printed in the United States of America

13/QGT-CML/1

CONTENTS

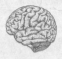

Chapter 1

▶ Sustain Your Brain 6

Chapter 2

▶ Changing the Forecast 28

Chapter 3

▶ Redefining Reality 42

Chapter 4

▶ A Body in Motion 64

Chapter 5

▶ Name That Tune 84

Chapter 6

▶ Attention, Please 104

Chapter 7

▶ Instant Replay 120

Chapter 8

▶ More Than Words 160

Chapter 9

▶ Take Charge 184

Chapter 10

▶ Live Smart 204

▶ Glossary 226

▶ Further Reading 230

▶ About the Author and the Consultant 233

▶ Index 234

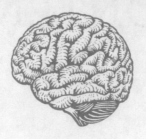

CHAPTER 1

Sustain Your Brain

Keeping your body's command center in peak condition

Your brain's health may be the most powerful indicator of how long you will live. It is crucial to whether that life will be rich and satisfying from youth well into old age, or something substantially less rewarding, and for less time.

A car driven wisely, fueled with high-quality gasoline, given regular oil changes, and repaired with new parts as old ones wear out is likely to last longer than one that's abused or neglected. Likewise, the easiest way to have a healthy brain in middle age and beyond is to start with one as a youth and to follow good physical and mental habits. Exercise it. Feed it. Challenge it. Then enjoy the rewards.

But what of the person who comes late to repairs, like the owner of a car that rusts for years on blocks or runs too long on dirty oil? The car owner can always swap out the engine. You, on the other hand, have only one brain, basically composed of the same neurons you were born with, plus a few added to some narrowly specific areas. Once they've begun to deteriorate, can they be saved—or even made stronger?

Brain researcher Marian Diamond is certain they can.

In the 1960s, Diamond compared two groups of lab rats. The first group was confined to the equivalent of a gray isolation cell in a maximum-security prison. They ate simple rations to keep them alive from day to day, but their brains received little stimulation. No rat games, no rat puzzles, no rat get-togethers to break the boredom. She enrolled the second group in a version of rat school, complete with recess. They had toys and balls for play, challenging mazes to explore, exercise equipment to get blood pumping to their muscles and their neurons, and best of all, other rats to share their experiences. When she pitted the two in timed contests in which they ran the same mazes, the rats that had lived in the mentally and physically invigorating environment performed much better.

▶ NEW KIND OF FITNESS REGIMEN
Learning can strengthen your brain at any age

Diamond then did what she could not do to humans in a similar experiment. She put both winners and losers under the knife to examine their brains. (Life's not fair, especially for rodents.) Rats that had enjoyed the richer learning environment and had won the maze races exhibited markedly different brains from those in the control group. Their cerebral cortices—the outer, wrinkled shells that are home to neural pathways that make sense of the world— were thicker than those of the unstimulated rats. The enriched-brain rats had more neural connections, a sign of greater mental activity. And they had more blood vessels to carry vital oxygen to keep those connections firing at peak efficiency. Diamond had gathered concrete evidence that what goes on in the mind manifests itself in the physical state of the brain. Learning strengthens the organ of the brain just as exercise strengthens muscles in the legs, arms, and abdomen.

As revealing as Diamond's research was, it had a twist: She didn't experiment on young rats. She chose to work with rats in middle age and older, equal to ages between 60 and 90 in humans. Old rats had brains they could reshape in response to new experiences, a condition known as plasticity.

Experience Is Everything

That revelation changed widespread beliefs about the plasticity of older brains. Studies with young rats, cats, and other mammals had

---

BRAIN BOOSTER

YOUR TOTAL BRAIN WORKOUT

Look for the "Brain Booster" boxes to find tested methods
for boosting brainpower

Although the research on brain health is still young, current science suggests that practicing good health habits across different aspects of well-being may be our best ticket to staying sharp and lowering our risk for dementia.

Throughout this book, you will find a series of tips and exercises based on the Total Brain Health® program, a unique approach to improving brain fitness that I have developed and taught to audiences and private clients. These exercises and tips give you scientifically grounded advice and activities that you can really use to practice better brain fitness in ways that engage your body, mind, and spirit. Use the Brain Booster to take the information you are learning here to the next level.

—Cynthia R. Green

suggested that the brain opened a crucial window for learning during youth, and then closed it. For instance, in a series of famous experiments in the 1960s, neurobiologists David Hubel and Torsten Wiesel took a group of kittens and sewed one of each pair of eyes shut at birth but left the other untouched. At six months, they opened the closed eye. Although the eye was physically sound, the kitten never learned to see through it.

The experiment demonstrated that the kitten's brain had been wired to expect, and process, visual information at a crucial time in development. When that time passed, those abilities were gone forever. Scientists call this type of brain development "experience-expectant," meaning the brain awaits the stimulus of a particular experience, such as sight or sound, to develop the means to process that information.

No Age Limits

But there's a second category of brain-developing experiences. These are called "experience-dependent." They prompt brain growth in response not to stimuli common to the species, such as light and sound, but rather to the individual's unique environment. A child raised in the Amazon jungle learns a lot about plants and animals of the rain forest. A child growing up in the suburbs figures out how to play on the jungle gym and swings, or to swim in a pool or kick a soccer ball.

This second type of brain development can occur at any time. Some types of learning, such as mastery of a second language, are easier before the age of puberty, but on the other hand, vocabulary building occurs throughout life. In general, there is no single, crucial time window for this kind of learning. Your brain can learn experience-dependent knowledge at any time.

▶ THE UNIVERSE INSIDE YOUR HEAD
Getting to know your body's most dynamic system

The brain's plasticity reveals much about its amazing structure. It is the most complicated object in the universe, composed of billions of independent units that work together in remarkably complex symphonies that manage to comprehend the world; process, store, and retrieve information; and use that information to decide how to interact with the world. Each new experience changes the brain's physical makeup, so that by the time you finish reading this page, your brain will be slightly different from your brain at the time you began with the page's first word.

At the cellular level, the human brain is a collection of as many as 100 billion nerve cells called neurons and about 50 trillion neuroglia cells. The latter sometimes are simply called glial cells, from the Greek word for "glue." Their role is similar to that of hordes of servants in a castle: They serve their comparatively few masters, the neurons. Glial cells help neurons make connections and promote their health and steady functioning. Some take an active role in physical health by attacking microbes. Others, called oligodendrocytes, produce an insulating substance called myelin that speeds communication from neuron to neuron.

Wired for Connectivity

Neurons are the brain's key players. Each begins as its own little orb. Once the neuron has fixed itself into its particular cubbyhole in the brain during fetal development, two types of projections sprout from its central core: a single, whiplike axon, some as short as a fraction of an inch and others several feet long, and from one to as many as 100,000 dendrites branching out like the knobby ends of a cat-o'-nine-tails. Dendrites reach out to other neurons, some near and some far. They receive information from the axons of their neighbors and pass it to their neuron for processing; their input allows a neuron to gather data—to learn. The neuron initiates or passes information via its axon to the dendrites of other neurons, like a teacher speaking to a classroom of students, with each of those students channeling the information to other students, parents, and friends. The web of axons and dendrites pointing in every direction makes the brain's interior wiring resemble the chaos of a mangrove swamp.

BRAIN INSIGHT

From Chaos to Cognition

As Emily Dickinson once wrote, "The brain is wider than the sky"

Your brain is astonishingly, incomprehensibly, jaw-droppingly complicated.

Assume that each of your brain's roughly 100 billion neurons (nobody has counted them, but that's a pretty good estimate) has the capability to connect with one to as many as 10,000 other neurons, thanks to its arrangement of axons and dendrites. If that's the case, then the number of theoretical connection patterns in your brain is 40 quadrillion: 40,000,000,000,000,000. If you factor in the variable power of how strongly neurotransmitters send a signal from one neuron to the next, hypothesizing that each neuron has ten different signal strengths, then the number of electrochemical configurations in the brain runs to ten to the one-trillionth power. That's the number 1, followed by a trillion zeros. Compare this with the estimates of the number of atoms in the observable universe: 10 to the 80th power, or 1 followed by 80 zeros.

Out of this mind-blowingly vast maze of neural connections of varying intensities comes the ability to comprehend and interact with the universe. At some point in the brain's development, consciousness arises within a three-pound, tofu-like mass of wrinkled matter. The universe becomes aware of itself—and can marvel at its own complexity.

▶ IT STARTS WITH A SPARK
Neural communication runs on electricity

If only you could watch as information passes along circuits of neurons, it might look like flocks of birds darting, converging, and scattering against the sky. Like birds in flight, reeling and turning as if by magic, neurons communicate without the need to touch one another. A tiny space, called a synapse, separates the would-be embrace of axons and dendrites.

The neuron's language of communication within its own cell body is electricity. A spark received via a dendrite travels as electric energy until it reaches the end of the neuron's axon. There, the information it contains is translated into a variety of chemicals known as neurotransmitters. Each neurotransmitter has its own particular job, ranging from energizing the receiving neuron to fostering positive feelings of rewarding behaviors to suppressing particular actions. The neurotransmitters traverse the synaptic gap and dock in matching receptor sites like keys in a lock. Their joining with the cell wall of the receptor neuron initiates a new electrical charge, which travels the length of *that* neuron until it is converted to chemical energy at the far side.

A neuron requires stimulation to fire. That stimulus could begin outside the body, as when you look at the sea and electromagnetic waves reflecting off the surface activate the light-sensitive rod and cone cells in your eyes' retinas. That sensation—blue or green, flat, rolling, or choppy—knocks down the first domino in the line. From the retina, the signal passes along a neural chain to the visual cortex at the back of the brain and then back to the front for further processing. A stimulus could also originate internally, as when you feel hungry, or when your conscious mind remembers the face of your fifth-grade teacher and activates the first neuron in another domino-like pattern.

BRAIN INSIGHT

The MVPs of Your Mind

These chemicals are some of the most important messengers in the brain

▶ **ACETYLCHOLINE.** Causes muscles to contract; also linked to memory, sleep, and attention.

▶ **DOPAMINE.** Crucial for movement of the body, as well as the brain's reward system, associated both with pleasure and addiction. Patients with Parkinson's disease have lowered dopamine levels, causing characteristic shaking of limbs and head.

▶ **ENDORPHIN.** Released following stress or pain, acting like a natural opiate by binding to opiate receptors on neurons.

▶ **GAMMA-AMINOBUTYRIC ACID, or GABA.** Quiets, rather than excites, neurons, because the brain needs to decelerate as well as accelerate a multitude of functions.

▶ **GLUTAMINE.** Excites neurons, except in high concentrations fatal to neurons; required for learning and memory.

▶ **NOREPINEPHRINE.** Plays a key role in regulating mood, as well as blood pressure, heartbeat, and arousal.

▶ **SEROTONIN.** Prompts sleep and appetite; also plays a role in mood, related to everything from depression to anxiety to sexual arousal.

Some neurons fire consciously, and some fire below the level of conscious thought. Some even fire in ways to mimic the world outside.

When a particular bit of information travels throughout a circuit of neurons, it changes from electrical to chemical, back and forth, propagating a signal at speeds that can reach more than two hundred miles an hour. As it travels, it may prompt the addition or subtraction of more information, or set off a flood of new signals with new information. All this motion requires energy. The brain accounts for only about 2 percent of a body's weight, but it uses about 25 percent of the body's blood sugar and oxygen.

Because neurons aren't bound to each other like bricks in a wall, they remain free to make new connections and break old ones. That's exactly what happens when the brain learns something new: The information physically alters the connections.

▶ PIECES OF A PUZZLE
Understanding your brain's anatomy

At the micro level, neurons in their billions form an intricate electrical net. At the macro level, they are organized into the discrete structures of the brain, with four main parts: cerebrum, diencephalon, cerebellum, and brain stem.

The outer surface of the cerebrum, nearest the skull, is the cerebral cortex. It's the wrinkly, gray, walnut-shaped covering that most people think of when they visualize the brain. The cerebral cortex is home to the functions of information processing that separate humans from other animals.

The cerebrum exists in two hemispheres, the left and right, connected by a band of neural tissue called the corpus callosum, which allows information to pass between the two. The left hemisphere has long been considered dominant because it typically is the site of language processing. Strokes in the left hemisphere sometimes impair speech. Injuries to the right hemisphere, on the other hand, sometimes result in reductions

SMALL STEPS TO BETTER BRAIN HEALTH

You need only a few minutes a day to build new brain connections

Sometimes making the change to better health can seem overwhelming. Where do you start? How can you fit it all in?

➡ **STEP 1: SMALL STEPS**
When it comes to your brain, even small steps can help you get on the road to better brain fitness. Look for small ways in which you can do something just a bit differently, such as taking a different route to work, learning a short meditation practice, or taking five minutes each day to study a poem. Such challenges offer us all the chance to wrap our minds around something in a slightly different way, forcing us to set new neural connections and pathways.

➡ **STEP 2: THINK DIFFERENTLY**
The Brain Boosters included here offer you many simple yet fun ways to change your brain game. They are designed to make it easier for you to bring better brain health into your daily routine.

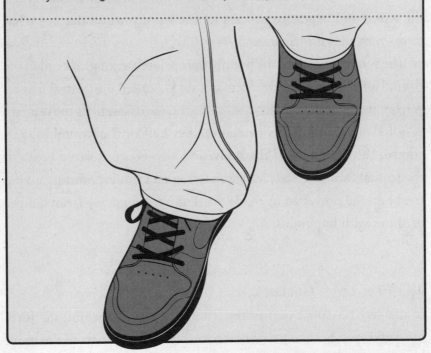

in or loss of the ability to integrate information—to see the forest for the trees. The right hemisphere apparently plays a crucial role in emotional and spatial recognition, such as seeing raised eyebrows and upturned corners of the mouth and realizing that a face expresses joy.

The two hemispheres duplicate many anatomical structures. Brain experts speak of folds and fissures dividing the hemispheres into four lobes, but each lobe has a separate left and right half. As a result, neurologists sometimes refer to a particular lobe in the singular or plural, but may be talking about the same thing.

▶ THE LOWDOWN ON YOUR LOBES
Functions of the front and back sections

In general, the back portion of the brain takes in information about the world and begins to process it. The front portion decides what to do with that information.

The foremost part of the brain, appropriately enough, is called the frontal lobe. It lies in front of a major divide called the central fissure. A frontal lobe region called the precentral gyrus controls movement. A quirk of evolution has caused the left half of the frontal lobe to control the right side of the body, and vice versa. Related areas of the frontal lobe oversee complex motion and inhibit motion, giving the brain the power to override the desire to run away from danger or shout with happiness.

The Prefrontal Cortex

In the very foremost part of the frontal lobe, right behind the forehead and eyes, lies the prefrontal cortex (PFC). This part of the brain developed last on the evolutionary time line, and is the last to become fully myelinated. The PFC is the region that most separates humans from all other animals, including apes. It comprises 30 percent of the human brain, compared with only 11 percent for a chimpanzee and 3 percent for a cat. It is the home of decision making and thus is sometimes called the brain's seat of "executive function"—it is the boss.

That Little Voice You Can't Ignore

Clinical neuroscientist Daniel G. Amen considers the boss metaphor apt. When the boss is absent in an office or factory, sometimes little serious work gets done, Amen says. And when the PFC boss works very hard, micromanaging the rest of the conscious brain, it sometimes promotes anxiety and worry—and again, little useful work gets done. Amen also likens the PFC to the Disney cartoon character Jiminy Cricket, who acted as the conscience of the puppet-boy Pinocchio. The cricket's still, small voice suggested the best ways to behave. When the guiding voice grows too quiet, the result is what Amen calls "Jiminy Cricket deficiency syndrome." Negative behaviors multiply, including impulsive action, confusion, short attention span, bad judgment, low empathy, poor time management, and diminished conscience.

Got That Feeling? It's All in Your Head

Behind the frontal lobe lie the parietal and temporal lobes. The parietal lobe processes sensations from the body, including pain and the pressure of touch. The temporal lobe processes sounds, including speech. It is also associated with memory and the emotional content of experiences. Each half of the temporal lobe includes a small, seahorse-shaped form called the hippocampus, which comes from the Greek words for "horse" and "sea monster." The hippocampus is part of the limbic system, a collection of structures on the inside of the cerebral cortex associated with emotions, motivation, and behavior.

▶ THE MIRACLE OF MEMORY
An internal filing system that never taps out

Neuroscientists once believed that the mature brain was incapable of producing new neurons—that the neurons you had at birth, or shortly afterward, were the only ones you would have for your entire life. Research in the 1990s laid that idea to rest. New neurons have been found growing in the hippocampus, a region that is crucial in the formation and storage of memories. In a famous study in 2000, University College London neuroscientist Eleanor Maguire demonstrated enlarged hippocampi in the brains of London cabdrivers. Cabbies spend two to four years memorizing London's intricate street grids, including the shortest distance between any two points. Using a magnetic resonance imaging (MRI) scanner, Maguire found that cabbies' right posterior hippocampus, a region devoted to spatial navigation, measured 7 percent larger than the norm. Evidently, neuroplasticity had reshaped the cabbies' brains as they learned more and more about navigating through London.

At the back of the brain is the occipital lobe. Although it is at the opposite end of the brain from the eyeballs, the occipital lobe processes visual information. Much of the lobe interprets shape, color, motion, and other qualities of objects sensed by the retinas of the eyes, which are extensions of the brain. This information-processing set of neural circuits is called the visual cortex.

BRAIN INSIGHT

It's Personal

A famous accident illustrated the connections between personality and parts of the brain

A gruesome accident in 1848 linked the prefrontal cortex to moral behavior. Vermont railroad worker Phineas Gage was jamming a tamping iron into a hole to pack gunpowder and sand when the iron sparked on a rock. The powder exploded, sending the 13-pound rod through Gage's cheek, prefrontal cortex, and skull crown. Gage initially seemed barely fazed. "Here is business enough for you," he told a doctor.

Before the accident, co-workers liked Gage and considered him reliable and temperate. After the accident, he became rude, impatient, profane, and unable to stick to plans. Gage drifted from job to job and died 12 years later, at 36, after a series of seizures.

In 2012, a team of researchers at UCLA's Laboratory of Neuro Imaging (LONI) published a paper tracing the path of the tamping iron through Gage's brain. They managed to produce a striking new image of the damage, while tracing the probable severed connections to other parts of his brain. They concluded that Gage's behavioral changes came not only from harm to his prefrontal cortex, but also from the disrupted pathways to other areas that involve emotional response—showing once again that the brain is an immensely interconnected organ.

► ALWAYS ON DUTY
The parts of your brain that drive you from day to day

Moving out of the cerebrum, the diencephalon lies between the left and right hemispheres. Its structures regulate body rhythms such as sleeping and wakefulness, as well as body temperature, digestion, perspiration, and other body functions that usually occur below the level of consciousness. A portion of the diencephalon known as the thalamus relays sensory information from other brain regions and plays a role in emotion and memory.

The Balancing Act

Below the occipital lobe is the cerebellum. Although it contributes to emotional life and action, the cerebellum's most obvious task is to coordinate movement and balance. The cerebellum automatically processes the neural signals required to perform practiced tasks. For

---

BRAIN INSIGHT

The Man Who Forgot

In 1953, time stopped passing for Henry Molaison, known to history as HM

Henry Molaison's troubles began early. He began having epileptic seizures as a child after a being hit by a bicycle in his native Connecticut. Whole-brain seizures increased in frequency until, by age 27, in 1953, he suffered nearly a dozen a week.

His doctor reasoned they would stop if he eliminated their point of origin, so he surgically removed much of Molaison's temporal lobes, including the left and right hippocampus. The operation indeed halted the seizures. But Molaison awoke without the ability to make new memories. The hippocampus turns out to be crucial to the transference of short-term memories into longer storage.

For the next 55 years, until he died in 2008, Molaison had the most-studied brain on the planet. Researchers repeatedly tested aspects of his memory, including the conscious and unconscious, the short and long term. Academic papers referred only to patient "HM" to preserve Molaison's privacy while he lived.

Molaison cheerfully submitted to every test; he never realized their endless repetition and could never get bored. If someone erased a crossword puzzle after he completed it, he happily did it—again and again. He lived in a permanent "now," thinking he was still 27, until the day he died.

example, when you learn to type, you concentrate to find and hit the right keys. That action, which initially requires focused attention and choices, takes place mostly in your frontal lobes. But as you grow comfortable with the location of the letters, you type without consciously thinking of where to find each key. Your cerebellum houses the autopilot that keeps the right keys clicking. Other brain regions jump into action to pay attention and recognize when you hit the wrong ones.

The fourth major brain region is the brain stem. It comprises the area where the brain meets the spinal cord, which is merely an extension of neurons into the body. Key brain stem regions include the medulla oblongata, which controls heartbeat and respiration, and the pons, which controls reflexes such as the startled jump you make when a door slams shut. Largely beyond conscious control, this lowermost portion of the brain is nevertheless crucial to survival.

▶ THE BIRDS AND THE BEES AND THE BRAIN
The humble origins of a powerful organ

The entire structure of the adult human brain lies hidden in the genetic code that begins to find expression at conception. When sperm slams into egg, uniting a father's and mother's DNA, the reaction causes the fertilized egg to begin dividing. At four weeks, the first brain structures begin to appear. A spoon-shaped neural plate takes shape at the head end of the developing body. A groove later appears in the center of the plate, and hemispheres begin to form on either side shortly after that. The spoon's bowl becomes the brain itself, and the handle transforms into the spinal cord. Major brain regions start to develop, with the cerebral cortex witnessing the most explosive growth.

About a quarter million neurons form *every minute* in the early months of fetal development, and migrate to particular regions of the brain to take up specialized tasks. Axons and dendrites sprout when the neuron arrives at its destination. Neuroscientists once believed neurons chose their favored sites because each new neuron already had a predetermined function and sought the site associated with that function. Now, scientists believe that the journey and the destination shape the neuron to perform one task or another.

Although the brain reacts to its environment at all times, the period of so-called "neuron migration" in the womb marks a high state of sensitivity. Serious consequences can result from toxins or anything else interfering with neurons as they move through the prenatal brain, causing them to fall short of or overshoot their destination. Dyslexia and autism, for example, have been linked, in part, to less-than-optimal neural migration. The brain's in utero sensitivity underscores the need for pregnant women to eat well, exercise, and avoid alcohol, tobacco, and other substances that could hinder the neural development of their children.

Survival of the Fittest (Neurons)

At eight months after conception, the fetal brain contains twice as many neurons as an adult's, even though the younger brain weighs only about one-third of the adult brain. The brain cannot sustain that many neurons and neural connections, so it begins to cut back. About half of the brain's neurons die in the final weeks of fetal development. In addition, many of the neural connections grow weak and dissolve, a process known as pruning. The result, at birth, is that the brain contains virtually all of the neurons it will have for life. Brains get bigger as the child ages into an adult for two reasons. First, the brain's neurons grow physically larger by sending out more dendrites. And second, supporting cells around the neurons, particularly the glial cells, multiply to increase the brain's total volume.

After birth, the newborn's brain undergoes a kind of neural Darwinism. Neural networks compete to have the strongest links, while weak links receiving little or no stimulation undergo rigorous pruning. A widely repeated adage about the brain says, "Use it or lose it." That appears to be literally true, especially when a child's brain, primed to react to virtually any stimulation, receives some kinds but not others.

BRAIN INSIGHT

Maximum Capacity

Sorry, but you're already using all of your brain

In the 2011 movie *Limitless*, a character played by actor Bradley Cooper takes a pill that supposedly allows him to call on the cognitive power of his entire brain, rather than the 20 percent that the movie says humans normally access.

University of Minnesota physics professor James Kakalios, author of *The Amazing Story of Quantum Mechanics*, concedes that taking certain drugs can boost brainpower in the short run. However, he considers taking a pill to become a genius to be "crazy," far, far beyond current neurochemistry's boundaries.

The movie also perpetuates the myth that the human brain uses only a small percentage of its neurons. "We use all of our brains," Kakalios told NBC. "We don't understand a lot about how the brain works, but evolutionarily, everything in the three-pound hunk of meat on the top of your head is there for a reason."

Brain-imaging technology reveals no dead spots in a healthy brain. Although neural plasticity allows the brain to reroute the pathways for some functions around dead or damaged cells, demonstrating that some neural regions sometimes can be circumvented without complication, no neurons take a free ride inside the skull. Every brain cell has its function.

BRAIN-HEALTHY LIVING IN TEN STEPS

What's good for your body and your social life is good for your brain, too

. . . .

Here's all you need to know in just ten steps:

➲ **STEP 1**
Get regular exercise.

➲ **STEP 2**
Eat a healthy, well-balanced diet and maintain a healthy weight.

➲ **STEP 3**
Stay on top of your health and use medications wisely.

➲ **STEP 4**
Get a good night's sleep, avoid risky behaviors, and don't stress!

➲ **STEP 5**
Play games against the clock to stay sharp and focused.

➲ **STEP 6**
Use simple memory strategies to enhance your daily recall.

➲ **STEP 7**
Keep your mind engaged through new challenges. Find little ways to "change up" your brain's routine.

➲ **STEP 8**
Be social—it offers great challenge for everyday thinking skills.

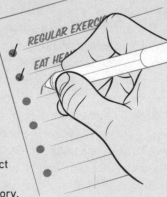

➲ **STEP 9**
Work or volunteer to stay intellectually challenged and socially engaged. Both activities may offer protection from memory loss over time.

➲ **STEP 10**
Think positively! Self-perception can affect our performance. Practice the power of positive thinking and believe in your memory.

▶ HEAD START
Harnessing youth's advantages

The younger the brain, the more plasticity it has. Not just language but virtually any skill is learned most easily when taught to a young brain. Thanks to his father's instruction, Tiger Woods, perhaps the greatest golfer in the history of the game, already had learned the fundamentals of the game at age two. Plasticity also makes its virtues evident when a child suffers a brain injury. Young brains have a greater capacity to rewire themselves to minimize or even eliminate the impact of a serious injury. The reason, according to University of Wisconsin neuroscientist Ronald E. Kalil, may be that youthful brains are bathed in growth-enhancing chemicals that assist the brain in reconstruction and reorganization. Kalil found these factors in young cats, whose brains repaired themselves efficiently, but found far less of them in less-responsive adult cat brains.

The Mechanics of Moodiness
The brain goes through a rocky phase in adolescence. It directs a physical body that resembles an adult's, but it has yet to complete its development. In particular, the foremost parts of an adolescent brain—the portion that controls behavior—usually have yet to complete myelination. That can lead to moody behavior (surprise!) as well as imperfect impulse control and other negative actions. A fully developed teenage cerebellum and motor cortex can direct a teen to smack a tennis serve into the opponent's court at 90 miles an hour. The impartially myelinated prefrontal cortex can also contribute to a temper tantrum if the teen double-faults on match point.

▶ THE TICKING CLOCK
Exploring the impacts of age

In the years from adolescence to old age, the brain continues to make new connections and prune underused ones. Aging brains shrink a bit as they lose some neurons and neural connections. A 90-year-old's brain typically weighs about 10 percent less than it did at its peak. The aging brain also begins to show changes in at least four important areas: speed of information processing, memory, neurons' inhibitory function, and sensation. Much of the decline occurs in the prefrontal cortex, as if the last part of the brain to be complete were the first to decline—a case of last in, first out. Variation in the species means that the brain can show signs of cognitive decline, affecting thinking and memory, at virtually any age. However, for many people, the first signs of slowing appear around age 50. The aging brain takes more time to learn new things and store them in memory. Meanwhile, the prefrontal cortex loses a measure of its ability to hold information in working memory, a sort of computer desktop where the brain keeps information at hand for immediate use. With the decline in long-term and working memory, the brain requires more time to store memories, retrieve them, and then make decisions based on them.

The brain's inhibitory function includes filtering out distractions. Too much information can make it difficult for the brains of typical people in their late 60s to figure out what's important and what's not. That can make driving difficult, as it requires discriminating between important traffic signs and unimportant ones. Or, elderly brains may experience sensory overload on busy metropolitan streets, but be OK on rural dirt roads.

Mature and elderly adults can still retain full plasticity to learn new tasks. Late in the 19th century, for example, people of all ages learned to ride bicycles when they made their appearance in the United States. Today, grandfathers of 70 and their granddaughters aged 2 can both learn how to use a tablet computer or smartphone.

STICK TO IT! STAYING WITH YOUR PLAN

Be realistic when you think through your brain health program

Changing our health habits can be hard. As any dieter can tell you, we start out committed, but easily find ourselves off track. Here are some tips for increasing the "stickiness" of your brain health plan:

➡ **SET A REALISTIC GOAL**
Make sure your goal is reachable. Remembering everything is unrealistic. Learning how to remember names is just the right size goal.

➡ **SET YOUR STRATEGY**
Figure out what steps you need to reach your goal. If improving name recall is your goal, decide whether you will take a course, read a book, or use some other technique. Break down your strategy into doable steps that are clear and easily accomplished.

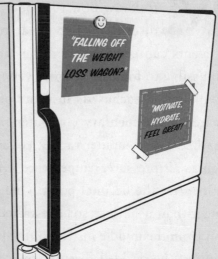

"FALLING OFF THE WEIGHT LOSS WAGON?"

"MOTIVATE, HYDRATE, FEEL GREAT!"

➡ **SET UP FOR SUCCESS— AND FOR FAILURE**
Plan the ways you can reward yourself as you move toward your goal. Everyone likes a pat on the back! At the same time, expect to hit some roadblocks. Figure out how you will get yourself back on track if you stray.

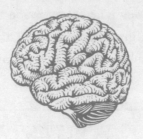

CHAPTER 2

....

Changing the Forecast

How to take brain health into your own hands

Meteorologist and mathematician Edward Lorenz wanted to know how to model weather patterns. Instead, he discovered two great truths: First, even the tiniest of events can generate enormous consequences; and second, it's impossible to forecast weather very far into the future.

At the Massachusetts Institute of Technology in 1961, Lorenz created a rudimentary computer program that simulated basic weather. The computer ran 12 equations to crunch weather data, such as air pressure, temperature, wind, and so on, that ran to six digits after the decimal point. One day, Lorenz wanted to run a longer-than-usual test, so he restarted a previous weather computation from the middle instead of the beginning. To make a compact printout, he decided to enter only the first three digits after the decimal point—representing his measurements to the thousandth part instead of the millionth. He figured that because he had made only the most minuscule changes to his input, the weather patterns would look the same.

Surprise. The new weather pattern veered dramatically away from the original. That fourth decimal place mattered. A lot.

Lorenz had discovered the roots of chaos theory. Science cannot measure everything, in infinite detail, that might affect a complex physical system. This means it is impossible to perfectly predict the system's performance in the future. Long-term meteorological forecasts fail because humans can never measure every variable, such as air temperature, down to the individual molecules of atmospheric gases. Nor can they predict when a particular unmeasured quality plays a crucial role in the system's performance.

▶ THE BUTTERFLY EFFECT
Small changes beget big outcomes

Lorenz's discovery has become known as the butterfly effect, after the title of his famous 1972 paper ("Does the Flap of a Butterfly's Wings in Brazil Set Off a Tornado in Texas?"). Most of the time, a butterfly flapping its wings doesn't alter weather patterns. But it can! Under the right conditions, the chain of events sparked by a butterfly fluttering or *not* fluttering its wings can lead to a storm.

Although weather is extremely complex, the human brain is ever so much more so. As a complex physical system, it too is subject to chaos theory. The tiniest thing can become its tipping point, leading to a significant, concrete change.

Tipping Points

It could tip for bad or good. Missing the bus to work by ten seconds might aggravate preexisting emotions enough for something truly bad to happen, such as causing you to get fired. Or, finding an Indian head penny in the dirt could lead to coin collecting as a new hobby, or drive away a dark mood and lead to a significant stretch of happiness. The decision to go for a walk around the block tomorrow morning before work, eat fresh fruit for breakfast, or do a crossword puzzle while waiting to see the dentist could signal the start of a new lifestyle that strengthens both body and brain.

The difference between the brain's bad and good tipping points is largely a matter of choice. Humans don't have the ability to stop bad things from happening. They can, however, use free will—the power to choose, embedded in the uniquely human prefrontal cortex—to opt to take steps to improve brain health. Chaos theory says the smallest step can lead to enormous alterations. You might do a brain exercise or two in this book and find yourself liking how you feel afterward. That may lead you to check out other mental or physical routines, within these pages or without. Before you know it, you've made a noticeable change in your mental circuitry. Your brain's plasticity ensures it will change as it makes new connections among your billions of neurons and even grows new brain cells in the hippocampus. Your free will makes you the engineer of those changes in your brain.

▶ GET PHYSICAL
Enhancing the mind-body connection

Your brain and body are connected by nerve bundles that move muscles and keep organs functioning. Nerves also provide sensory

STRIKE A BALANCE
Bring your "weaker" side up to par

A key component of coordination and balance can be the degree to which we have evenness, or symmetry, of ability across both sides of our body. Most of us have dominance on either the left or right side. We favor that side, hand, or foot when we do things such as write, play sports, or perform other tasks that require fine motor dexterity and coordination. Yet what about your other half? Doesn't it need to stay in the game?

➡ A GREAT WAY to challenge our nondominant side and encourage better balance is through activities that ask us to coordinate and engage both sides of our brain at the same time. Hobbies like knitting, playing instruments such as the piano or violin, or juggling do just that.

Take some time to figure out how you can better strike a balance by challenging yourself with exercises that get both sides of your body on par. You may find your nondominant side slower and less agile at first, but keep up the work!

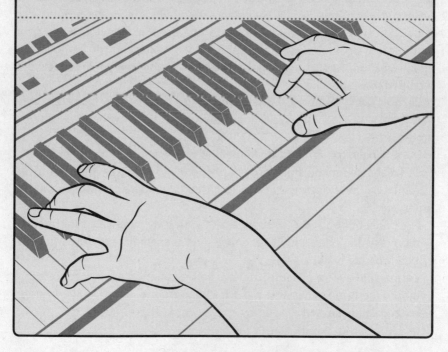

stimuli from your body for your brain to process. It should be no surprise, then, that a healthy brain begins with a healthy body. Recognition of the mental–physical relationship dates at least to ancient Rome, which gave us the Latin phrase *Mens sana in corpore sano* ("A sound mind in a healthy body").

BRAIN INSIGHT

A Walk in the Park

Sometimes, helping your brain may be as simple as a walk in the park

M arc Berman, a postdoctoral fellow at Toronto's Rotman Research Institute, found that walking for an hour improved cognitive function and mood among adults diagnosed with clinical depression.

Berman recruited 20 clinically depressed subjects in and around Ann Arbor, Michigan, and assigned them to two groups. The first walked for an hour in a peaceful woodland setting and the second for an hour in a noisy urban setting. A week later, the two groups switched venues and repeated the experiment.

Berman was skeptical: People with depression often seize on dark thoughts, and a solitary walk might give them time to focus on painful times in their lives.

Surprisingly, the 2012 study found that walkers in both settings experienced a boosted mood. Furthermore, those in the natural setting improved attention and working memory by 16 percent compared with those in the urban setting.

The study built upon a 2008 experiment that demonstrated that people without any diagnosis of illness enjoyed increased memory and attention after a woodsy walk.

Berman believes a peaceful, natural setting eliminates distractions that bombard the brain's memory and attention circuits, allowing the brain to relax and restore itself.

Getting to the Heart of the Matter

Many brain health programs begin by focusing on the body's physical health. The brain's around-the-clock work schedule consumes a quarter of all the blood the heart circulates. The stronger the pumping heart, the more efficient the functioning of the brain. Having a healthy heart requires a proper diet, low in fat and high in fiber and antioxidants, as well as a regimen of regular exercise and abstention from dangerous toxins such as those in tobacco and illegal drugs.

Any kind of exercise is better than none. Walking, swimming, dancing, biking . . . whatever elevates your pulse and gets you sweating improves the function of your heart and lungs, sending life-giving oxygen to your neurons. Exercise has been found to reduce the risk of heart attack, diabetes, and colon cancer, and also beneficially affects blood pressure and mood. But exercise also physically changes the brain. Aside from boosting the amount of oxygen red blood cells carry to the neurons, exercise increases the density and number of blood vessels in the motor cortex and cerebellum, which control conscious and unconscious movement. True exercise is the key—you can't boost the amount of oxygen to your brain simply by speeding your breathing patterns. Deliberately trying to hyperventilate, by taking fast and shallow breaths, actually decreases oxygen levels in the brain. Cerebral hypoxia, or low levels of brain oxygen, can cause fainting.

Know Your Enemies

In addition to heart and artery disease and lack of exercise, factors that limit the flow of blood to the brain include:

▶ **Nicotine.** Smoking cuts the flow of blood to every organ, and the brain is no exception.

▶ **Dehydration.** No surprise here: The brain is 80 percent water. When starved for water, it staggers to perform physical functions and struggles to focus attention.

▶ **Caffeine.** Not only does it directly reduce blood flow, but it also can disrupt sleep and cause dehydration. On the other hand, some evidence suggests benefits to the brain from the daily stimulus of a measured amount of caffeine in coffee or tea. For example, caffeine improves attention, which is essential to learning and memory.

▶ **Lack of sleep.** Studies have shown that people who sleep less than six hours per night have decreased blood flow to the brain. As anyone would know when getting out of bed after a fitful night of tossing and turning, a poor night's sleep also impairs memory, mood, and overall cognitive function.

▶ **Drug and alcohol abuse.** Drugs and alcohol have a toxic effect on vessels that carry blood and other bodily fluids. Like caffeine, however, red wine may have some benefits for the brain—not because of its alcohol content, but rather because of an ingredient called resveratrol that protects blood vessels.

▶ **Other toxins.** Many environmental poisons damage blood vessels.

▶ **Diabetes.** The disease causes blood vessels to grow brittle and interferes with proper healing of damaged tissue. It also increases risk of stroke.

▶ **Stress.** When the body reacts to potential danger, whether real or imagined, the endocrine glands prepare it for "fight or flight"—to supercharge it for combat against an enemy or predator, or to prepare it to run away. The flood of the stress hormone adrenaline shunts blood to the muscles at the expense of other regions.

WEAR YOUR WATCH UPSIDE DOWN

Small changes in familiar sights can exercise your brain

→ TODAY'S TIP WILL MAKE TIME FLY
Give your brain a little stretch each time you check your watch by wearing your watch upside down. This subtle change won't take much effort, but will force your brain to think out of its comfort zone in making sense of time gone a bit topsy-turvy. This is a great exercise for your visual perceptual skills, as you are forced to reinterpret familiar information in an unfamiliar way. Exercises like this, sometimes called "neurobics" (a phrase coined by Dr. Lawrence Katz), may seem fun and simple, yet are a terrific way to challenge our brain's flexibility and routine.

Like this exercise? Keep it going for a few more days.

Have a good time!

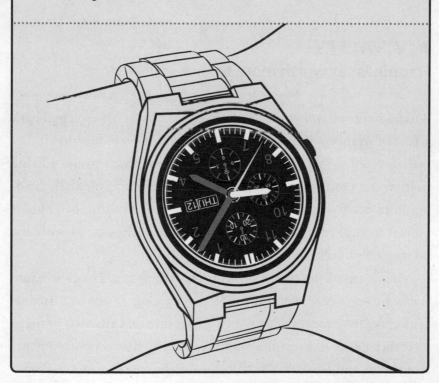

A small amount of stress can spark the brain to higher achievement, but stress that's too intense or chronic can damage the brain through changes in blood flow and pressure. Spikes in pressure caused by adrenaline can leave blood vessels vulnerable to breaking, which can be catastrophic in the brain. In addition to adrenaline, the stress hormone cortisol appears to impair memory. Studies of elderly adults demonstrated that those with high cortisol levels from long-term exposure to stress did worse on memory tests than similar adults with low levels of cortisol. The high-cortisol group also had smaller hippocampi, the brain region most closely associated with integration of memories. Children who experience prolonged exposure to high-stress environments also have trouble concentrating and learning.

▶ VITALITY
Happiness is worth more than a smile

Besides improving physical health, exercise boosts self-esteem. That's a part of vitality, another major component of brain health. Vitality includes feeling that your life has meaning, and that you enjoy living it. It means handling the storms and sunshine of life, mentally holding both positives and negatives in balance. A healthy social life is crucial to vitality, whether found in a circle of friends, co-workers, relatives, a church, or a community group.

Moods arise from chemical reactions in the brain. They also cause the brain to release chemicals that affect mood. It can be a vicious cycle. Negative mental states such as depression cause the brain to alter its balance of neurotransmitters in a way that supports a negative mood and interferes with brain functions. The mood-altered brain then mechanically releases even more chemicals linked to depression. Unchecked, this cycle can lead to isolation from a social circle (which usually enhances depression), and correlates with higher risk of dementia. On the other hand, happiness releases brain chemicals that benefit both brain and body even after the moment of joy passes. Laughter truly is a form of medicine.

Brain Food

Introspective techniques such as meditation can improve vitality and increase brain health. But you don't have to be a yogi to boost your inner peace. Because brain and body are so closely connected, you are, in part, what you eat, reinforcing the body's mental–physical relationship. Take fish, for example. A diet rich in fish and shellfish has been shown in multiple studies to keep the mind sharp and lower the risk of certain brain disorders. Residents of Iceland, who eat about five times as much seafood as Americans and Canadians, rarely have depression. Fish oil and, in particular, omega-3 fatty acids have been linked not only to brighter mood but also more efficient transmission of electrochemical signals between the synapses. Eating more fish may even raise the brain's shields to fight the onset of dementia.

▶ WORK IT OUT
Cognitive fitness arises from a range of activities

Along with physical health and vitality, a healthy brain requires something known as cognitive fitness. It's a measurement of the brain's functioning in four arenas: perception, attention, thinking, and language. All respond to the stimuli of new, complex activities by sprouting tangled thickets of axon-dendrite connections. The greater the complexity and novelty, the more the brain responds by making its internal connections even more complex.

Enhanced brain fitness has value in its own right. It feels satisfying at any age when you demonstrate mental agility and speed, as when you answer the questions while watching a game show on television or solve clever puzzles in the Sunday newspaper. But there's another, long-term benefit to engaging in brain-challenging games and activities: They raise your chances of maintaining your cognitive skills into old age. It appears that having a "brain reserve" of extra neural connections may provide a buffer against mental and physical decline with age.

Some loss is inevitable. The average human brain weighs about 1,400 grams, or roughly three pounds, at age 30. By age 90, the brain has lost 90 to 100 grams. The drop could be the result of neural death, loss of axon–dendrite connections that shrink neurons' weight, or both. Still, a popular theory posits that complexly wired brains have greater ability to hold on to their cognitive skills with advancing age. If something affects a number or percentage of neurons, it will have more impact on brains that are less fit and that have fewer neural connections. Richly wired brains still suffer neural losses, but they'll cope by shifting cognitive tasks to the web of neurons that remains.

The Brain Bank

A cognitive reserve acts like a savings account tapped on a rainy day to pay unexpected bills, which would break the bank of someone without the extra money. To use a computer example, imagine two brains as two internal hard drives. One brain, which has undergone fitness

ARTFUL ORIGAMI

Create original origami and stretch your visual imagination

The ancient Asian art of origami is a wonderful way to exercise your visual problem-solving skills and your imagination. Here, we are going to try a twist on the classic form of origami—instead of providing you with directions to fold and shape something specific, you are going to set out and use your mind and your creativity to see what you can come up with on your very own.

➔ FOLD IT FREESTYLE

Take a blank, square piece of paper of any size. Next, try folding it in many different ways (there is no right or wrong option in this exercise). Have fun as you fold, and see which shapes you can create along the way.

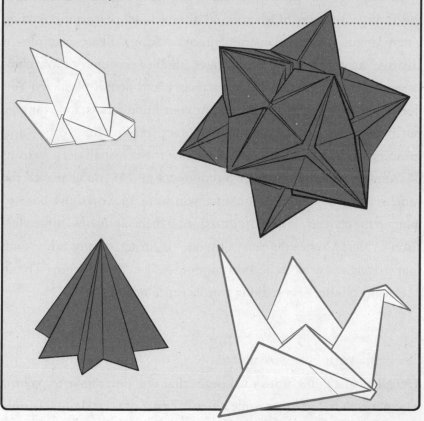

training, has added the equivalent of a supplementary memory, such as a flash drive or CD-ROM reader and stack of computer disks. When the enhanced computer loses its supplementary memory, its hard drive still functions. The loss may not even be noticeable. Such appeared to be the case with a study of nuns in Mankato, Minnesota, whose shared lifestyle made them ideal subjects. The nuns who had developed neurally enhanced brains through a lifetime of challenges appeared to keep their cognitive skills longer than those whose brains had less cognitive fitness. Sometimes, an autopsied nun's brain revealed the physical signs of Alzheimer's disease, even though the nun showed no evidence of Alzheimer's while alive.

Just as the body grows stronger when its muscles are challenged, the brain grows more fit when taxed by new kinds of learning. Adding a new language, musical instrument, or cooking skill are examples of creative categories of brain challenges. Smaller versions of those challenges work, too, thanks to chaos theory and neural plasticity. You don't have to learn Italian to enhance your brain fitness, for example, but if you're an opera buff, you might try learning the words—and meaning—of the soaring "Nessun dorma" ("None shall sleep!") from Giacomo Puccini's *Turandot*. Not an opera fan? If you've played the same six chords on the guitar since you were 15, you don't have to take up the clarinet. Instead, try mastering the melody of George Harrison's "Here Comes the Sun" on your six-string, or any other song that stretches your skills beyond your old limits. Always enjoyed basic Mexican cooking? Try making a *mole* sauce next time.

Unleash Your Inner Athlete

The glory of a good brain workout is that you don't have to pay for a gym membership or set aside a regular part of your daily schedule to take part. Many of the brain fitness activities explained in these pages can be done in just a few minutes, virtually anywhere and at any time.

If you want to go beyond the suggestions in this book, many games are available online, and software packages designed specifically to build skills, such as short-term memory, or build a reserve through intellectual engagement, such as learning a new instrument or traveling, are offered for purchase by a variety of manufacturers.

BRAIN INSIGHT

The Homer Simpson Gene

Could evolution have selected for a gene that makes us stupider?

Normally, when a gene is disabled or mutated, bad things result. However, knocking out a mouse gene known as RGS14 actually increases the mouse's ability to learn and remember information. A protein produced by the gene is believed to play a crucial role in the creation of memories, but strangely, when the gene is deleted in genetically altered mice, they get better at remembering and recognizing objects, easily recalling locations to help them speed more quickly through water mazes.

Pharmacologist John Hepler and colleagues at Emory University are so confident that RGS14, also found in humans, lowers brain performance that they have nicknamed it the "Homer Simpson gene," in honor of the cognitively challenged cartoon character. Mice without the gene created long-term, strong connections among neurons in the CA2 region of the hippocampus.

This raises what Hepler calls a big question: Why would evolution select for a gene that makes the brain less smart?

"I believe that we are not really seeing the full picture," he said. "RGS14 may be a key control gene in a part of the brain that, when missing or disabled, knocks brain signals important for learning and memory out of balance."

Further in the future are potential studies of the gene's impact on performance of the human brain.

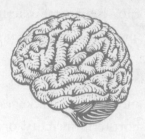

CHAPTER 3

Redefining Reality

Appreciating the brain as your window to the world

The relationship between the world "out there" and the brain's construction of it "in here" has fed centuries of highfalutin debate. In the 17th century, British philosopher John Locke argued that the brain passively processed information it collected about the world through the five senses. The German Immanuel Kant responded by proposing that the brain played a more active role, constructing the reality that humans navigate every day. Although the world has an underlying reality, he said, humans can never know it directly. Instead, all they have is the brain's constructed stage set of the world, with sights and sounds independent of the things they represented. A third philosopher, a contrary Irish theologian named George Berkeley, took things even further. He said there is no "real" world. To Berkeley, nothing existed without its being perceived by the brain through the senses. That idea seemed a bit much, not only to wags who wondered where the world went when it wasn't being perceived, but also to the British lexicographer and essayist Samuel Johnson, who kicked a rock and proclaimed, "I refute it thus!"

► MAKING SENSE OF YOUR SENSES
Perceptions arise from an integrated system

Their debate sheds light on the importance of a healthy brain and healthy senses. The nerves that sense light, sound, smell, taste, and touch are nothing but extensions of the brain. Without the optic nerve and light-sensitive retina, as well as the nerves that stretch and contract the muscles that cause the eye to blink, change focus, and shift its gaze, the brain would have no information to process in the visual cortex. So, questions about whether problems such as declining vision or hearing are matters of the eye or ear, or rather of the brain, are moot. The senses and the brain act as an integrated system, mixing perception and reality beyond the ability to separate them.

Time Takes Its Toll

The aging process changes the way sensory nerves send information to the brain. All senses become less acute at some point, causing the brain to have greater difficulty distinguishing details. This occurs for a variety of reasons, but two are paramount. First, the minimum amount of information required to register on the senses, called a threshold, increases with age. It takes more sound or more light, for example, to cause sensory nerves to fire, sending electrical signals to the brain. Second, changes in the sense organs themselves effect changes in perception. Alterations in organs and nerves associated with vision and hearing typically have the greatest impact, as sight and sound bear the greatest burden of constructing a mental map of the world that's useful for walking, driving, working, and other important activities. But changes in smell, taste, and touch shouldn't be dismissed. A world without pleasant scents and delicious food would lose much of the flavor of life; a world without appreciation of a soft breeze or a lover's caress also would feel diminished.

▶ OUT OF FOCUS
Searching for the source of vision problems

Many vision problems have nothing to do with aging. Myopia, or difficulty in seeing things at a distance, has become increasingly prevalent in the last few decades. It typically starts in childhood. In the United States, myopia rates have increased by two-thirds since the 1970s, a period that correlates to the introduction and diffusion of computers in the home and workplace. Theories that blamed computer monitors and other screens for the apparent epidemic emerged and gained popularity. A study of Alaskan Inuit seemed particularly compelling: They had few cases of myopia until television came to their homelands in the extreme north, when the number of cases zoomed.

However, a 1996 myopia study found no smoking gun. It said computers were no more likely than other forms of long-term, close-in work, such as reading, to be associated with myopia. The strongest indicator of a person's likelihood to develop nearsightedness, according to a 2007 study of California third graders, is heredity. Rates doubled if a child had one myopic parent and quintupled if he or she had two.

In the Dark

A more recent study, conducted by visual disorder expert Kathryn Rose of the University of Sydney, pointed to lack of exposure to sunlight as a possible contributing factor. Sunlight boosts dopamine levels in the brain, she found, in a way that fights the development of nearsightedness. The threshold for seeing benefits from sunlight seems to be 10 to 14 hours of exposure each week, she said. Slavish devotion to computers, television, and books may be linked to myopia merely because it tends to keep people indoors.

However, evidence remains plentiful for the connection between close work and something called "transient myopia," which is the bleary vision associated with long periods of reading. It results from the eyes' constant focus on a near plane. The condition won't cause permanent myopia, but it's an inconvenience in a world that relies so heavily on reading. The strain of prolonged attention to a computer screen also causes stress. It can cause eyes to go dry (from lack of blinking), and result in headache and muscle pains in the neck and shoulders. Once the symptoms of eyestrain appear, sufferers can try closing their eyes and rubbing their temples to feel better, or to improve reading conditions by increasing text size on a computer screen and adjusting ambient light.

▶ HOW TO STAY SHARP
Exercising for better eyesight

The eyes operate through muscle contractions. Exercise strengthens the muscles surrounding the eyes and helps keep their lenses flexible. Computer users in particular should take short breaks throughout the day to exercise their eyes. Exercises have been shown not only to help maintain a current level of vision but also to improve vision among people 65 and older.

Your Ocular Workout Plan

Eye exercises include the following, all of which should be accompanied by regular breathing to supply oxygen to the eyes, and blinking to keep the eyeball surface moist:

- ▶ **Palming.** This exercise, done without glasses or contact lenses, reduces stress. Sit at a table, lean forward, and put your left hand over your left eye so the heel rests on the cheekbone, the fingers lie flat on the forehead, and the cup of your palm covers but does not touch the eye. Then place your right hand over your right eye in the same manner, with your right-hand fingers on top of your left-hand ones. Keep your eyes open, and blink often. This technique relaxes both mind and eyes.
- ▶ **Tracking figure eights.** Visually trace a reclining figure eight, in the shape of the infinity symbol, about ten feet in front of you. Reverse the pattern once in a while.
- ▶ **Switching focal length.** Put your finger a few inches in front of your eyes. Focus on the finger, then focus on something in the distance beyond it. Switch back and forth.
- ▶ **Zooming.** Hold your thumb at arm's length. Focus your eyes on it as you bring your thumb close to your face, and move it back again.

Vision relies on neural networks in the brain. Like other neurons, they require stimulation to remain strong. "Use it or lose it" applies

BRAIN BOOSTER

EYE OPENER

Experience the world in a new way with just one eye

We rely on our visual perception to make sense of all that we see daily. Shouldn't we give it a good workout every once in a while?

➲ **FIVE-MINUTE CHALLENGE**
Try this simple exercise for at least five minutes each day (or in shorter sessions spread over the day) to challenge your visual perceptual capacity: Take a bandana, kerchief, or removable eye patch and use it to cover one eye. Keep that one eye covered and go about your regular routine. See how well you can see with just that one eye. What changes about your perception? Next, cover the other eye and see how things change.

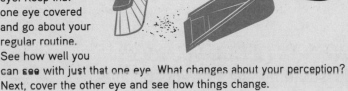

When you first start this exercise, try doing it while seated. If you do decide to move around, be sure to clear your path beforehand and avoid anything you might trip over. Keep in mind that your depth perception will be challenged, so move slowly and with care.

to seeing as much as it does to other brain activities. This was demonstrated by a study in 2010, in which test subjects improved their vision with the use of brain-challenging exercises.

Letters and Lines

A research team at the University of California, Riverside, and Boston University found that a specific set of eye exercises could clarify vision for a test group aged 65 and older. Subjects were shown a series of visual stimuli consisting of a letter embedded amid a field of horizontally oriented lines. The stimulus also included an array of peripherally located lines, in a diagonal orientation, that formed a vertical or horizontal object, and that always appeared in the same quadrant. Immediately after flashing an image, the researchers put up a masking pattern. The test subjects had to identify the central letter and peripheral object. Thus, their task was to perceive and process a confusing image in an instant. Two days of training in one-hour sessions with difficult stimuli prompted older subjects to substantially improve their vision, said chief researcher G. John Anderson. The improvement, related to physical changes in the visual cortex, lasted up to three months.

▶ WHY IS IT ALL BLURRY?
Understanding age's effects on eyesight

Around age 40, most adults start to experience an age-related decline in their ability to see things clearly at short distances, a condition known as presbyopia. It manifests itself gradually, but eventually causes difficulty in reading print. Those with the condition may find themselves "playing trombone," zooming a handheld page in and out until the eyes can bring it into focus. People who are already nearsighted sometimes find they have better close-in vision when they remove their eyeglasses. Some get two pairs of glasses, for near and distance vision, whereas others choose a single pair of bifocals or multifocals.

MIRROR, MIRROR
Challenge your mind with reverse perceptions

Here's a great way to reflect on the power of your perception.

➔ **LIFE IN REVERSE**
Place a small- to medium-size mirror in front of your keyboard or workspace. Then work a few minutes every hour or so while looking in the mirror, so that your actions are reversed. You can also try this when doing the dishes (make sure it's OK if the mirror gets splashed), writing, or doing other tasks where you can study your reflection.

Have young ones around? Mirror, Mirror is a great exercise to do with kids as well. Try it with them as they tie their shoes, do homework, or even color. It will bring about giggles but also some keen observations about what can happen when our visual perception is flipped.

This shift in your visual perception will definitely challenge how your brain usually sees the world.

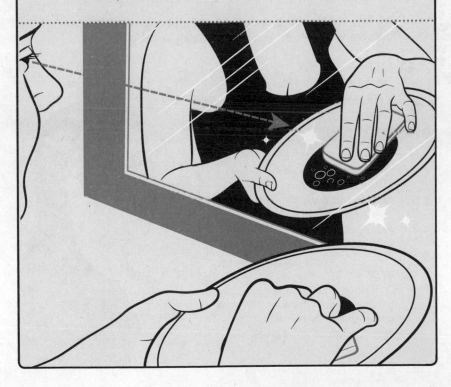

Presbyopia occurs as the lens—a transparent, flexible structure behind the iris—grows more rigid. The condition cannot be prevented or cured. It typically gets gradually worse, requiring changes in eyeglass prescriptions every two years or so, until about age 60, when it grows more stable.

Other conditions associated with aging of the visual system include the need for more light—to compensate for nerves' rising threshold—to read and perform other tasks; blurred vision and changes in the perception of color, especially blues and greens, as the

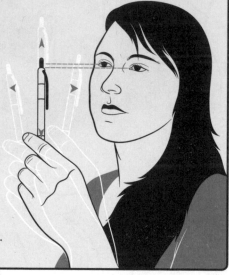

BRAIN BOOSTER

STAY FOCUSED!
Strengthen those eyes with a little exercise

Try this simple exercise designed to give your visual coordination a workout. All you need is a pen or pencil:

➜ **STEP 1**
Staring straight ahead, with your head level, hold a pencil with the eraser side up in your hand.

➜ **STEP 2**
Next, bring the pencil's end to eye level, and move the pencil from side to side, toward and away from your face, up and down, all while tracking the eraser with your eyes. Remember to keep your head still!

➜ **STEP 3**
Do this for a minute at first, building to about five minutes total each day (broken into several sessions if you prefer).

lens becomes cloudy and the cornea grows flatter; reduced production of tears, especially in postmenopausal women; greater incidence of glare, caused by the less-flexible lens scattering light on the retina instead of focusing it sharply; and pupils dilating less in low light.

BRAIN INSIGHT

The Proper Glasses, Always Ready
Ben Franklin's resourceful answer to presbyopia

Benjamin Franklin wore glasses for much of his life. As he aged, he had trouble not only with a general loss of visual acuity, but also a more pronounced blurriness when he looked at nearby objects.

The latter condition, called presbyopia, begins to affect many people around age 40. Unlike astigmatism, nearsightedness, and farsightedness, which arise from environmental and genetic factors reshaping the eyeball, presbyopia stems from the slow thickening and stiffness of the eyes' lenses with the passing of the years.

The 18th-century solution to Franklin's problem was to switch between two pair of glasses: one for reading, and one for general vision.

Franklin tried that for a while but thought better of it. "Finding this change troublesome, and not always sufficiently ready, I had the glasses cut and half of each kind associated in the same circle," he wrote. "By this means, as I wear my spectacles constantly, I have only to move my eyes up or down, as I want to see distinctly far or near, the proper glasses being always ready."

Although he may not have invented bifocals (historians argue the point), he was among the first to wear them, and he popularized them in the United States.

Bright Ideas for Preserving Vision
Compensation strategies allow many people to cope. Some may find it too difficult to drive at night, but will be perfectly comfortable

behind the wheel in daytime. Older people may use a red light in a darkened room, instead of a frosted-white or clear-bulb night-light, to reduce glare and may make a room more visible at night. Or they may adjust for the brain's lowered ability to distinguish blues and greens by decorating with more discernible reds, oranges, and yellows. Bright, warm colors make good accents not only on walls and furniture but also in pillows and afghans, which stimulate vision and sense of touch. These substitutions may help avoid bumps and bruises.

▶ GOOD VIBRATIONS
Hearing starts with a sound in your ear

Ears transform the vibrations of sound to electrical impulses that the brain can interpret in meaningful ways. The process begins when sounds collected by the outer ear travel to the eardrum, a thin flap of tissue that separates the outer ear from the middle ear, and set it to vibrating. High-pitched sounds make it vibrate more quickly than low ones, while loud sounds move the surface greater distances in and out. Each sound's distinct vibrations are passed through a succession of three tiny bones—the hammer, anvil, and stirrup—and wind their way to the inner ear. There, they strike tiny hairs growing in the cochlea, a snail-shaped organ that plays perhaps the most crucial role in hearing. The hairs transform the vibrations into electrical impulses, the only form of communication that can be read by the brain, and forward them along the auditory nerve.

The eardrum automatically grows more rigid in the presence of loud, low sound, which offers some protection against neural damage. But it remains vulnerable to sounds that blast too loud or last

REFRESH YOUR DRIVING SKILLS

Software can keep your mind and hands nimble

Keeping your eyes and your mind on the road are critical to staying safe while driving. Keeping our brain's focus, reaction time, and nimbleness up to speed as we grow older can be part of maintaining good driving habits and, for many older adults, our ability to stay independent and care for ourselves.

➜ GO FOR A VIDEO DRIVE

Take your brain for a test drive using a software program that reinforces the brain skills underlying good driving. There are several on the market: You might even find discounts or free versions through your auto insurance company. Find one that gives your attention, visual processing, reaction time, and flexibility a real workout. When you've found the one that suits you, make it a habit to spend some time each week tuning up your brain. It's a habit worth getting revved up about!

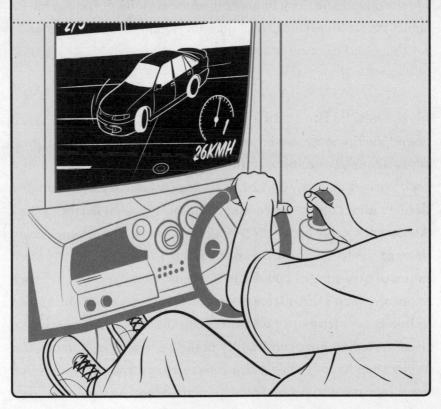

too long. Such sounds can weaken and even kill the sensitive hair cells in the cochlea. Once those cells are damaged or dead, they cannot be repaired or replaced. Cochlear implants bypass the hair cells by converting sounds into electrical impulses that directly stimulate the auditory nerve, but the implant-induced sensations lack the richness of natural sound. To maintain optimal hearing, it's best to avoid exposure to loud sounds, or to use protective ear wear if such exposure cannot be helped.

How much noise is too much? It depends on the loudness of the sound as well as duration of exposure. A single, powerful impulse, such as an explosion next to the head of a soldier in combat, can be enough to cause a condition called noise-induced hearing loss. On the other hand, long hours of moderately loud music can have a similar effect. In general, the louder the sound the less time it takes for the sound to cause serious damage.

How Loud Is Too Loud?

Sound energy is measured on the decibel scale. A whisper measures about 20 decibels, normal conversation about 60, and a rock concert as many as 120. It's a logarithmic scale, making 40 decibels about one hundred times as intense as a 20-decibel sound. An instant's exposure to the 140-decibel whine of a jet engine can damage the hair cells of the cochlea, but so too can two constant hours of exposure to 100 decibels. Hearing may return after such exposure, but it's often accompanied by a ringing or buzzing known as tinnitus. A lifetime of such ear damage can add up to a permanent decline. Audiologist Scott Bradley of the University of Wisconsin at Whitewater likens cochlear hair cells to a lawn and the sounds that wash over them to people walking on the grass. A single stroll over the lawn won't hurt it, but frequent travel will cut bare pathways.

Music lovers may not be aware of the potential for damage, despite warnings since the 1980s about portable music players equipped with headphones. More recent technology, which fits earbuds into the exterior opening of the ear canal, has only increased the risk.

"We're seeing the kind of hearing loss in younger people typically found in aging adults," said Dean Garstecki, a Northwestern University audiologist. He partly blames in-ear earphones, which can boost sound intensity by six to nine decibels. Garstecki's advice: To protect your ears, turn down the music.

BRAIN INSIGHT

Turning It Up to Eleven
The unwanted legacy of rock and roll

"Tommy, can you hear me?" Pete Townshend of the Who wrote those lyrics for his 1969 rock opera, *Tommy*, about a boy unable to see, hear, or speak.

It's also a question that hits home for Townshend, who lost much of his hearing after a lifetime of performing and recording loud rock music. Now in his late 60s, Townshend relies on two hearing aids, and according to a bandmate must stand next to the speakers to hear any of the music.

For a while, the Who held the world record for the loudest concert, a 1976 affair in London where the music topped 120 decibels. Other bands have broken that mark, and many other rockers have suffered hearing loss.

But Townshend puts primary blame on wearing earphones for studio work, and not concerts, for his decline. Prolonged exposure to loud music in earphones and their modern iPod cousin, earbuds, can damage hearing. One study at Wichita State University found students experiencing 110 to 120 decibels during normal earbud use. Constant exposure to 100 decibels can cause damage in two hours.

Diet for Better Hearing

Diets rich in antioxidants appear to strengthen neurons in the brain's auditory system against noise-induced hearing loss. Antioxidants neutralize free radicals, which damage neurons, including those that sense and process sound. Studies conducted in 2004 on Marines undergoing rifle training in California suggested that boosting the amount of antioxidants in their diet could lessen the effects of later exposure to loud battlefield noises—and possibly even help protect their cochlear hair cells if the antioxidants were ingested immediately after hearing extreme sounds. About 10 percent of Marines typically suffer some hearing loss as a result of rifle training. Now, daily doses of a drink that tastes like herbal tea and contains the supplement N-acetylcysteine, or NAC, may help them maintain their hearing.

▶ COULD YOU REPEAT THAT?
Why hearing becomes more difficult over time

Other forms of hearing loss occur naturally with age. The eardrum thickens and becomes more rigid, making it less sensitive to soft and high-frequency sounds. The ability to hear high-frequency sounds weakens more and more with age, with men older than age 70 experiencing hearing loss the most at the highest frequencies. Speech encodes vowel sounds in the lower range and consonant sounds in the higher range. As consonants carry more of the information of speech than vowels, high-frequency sound impairment can interfere with speech comprehension. That, in turn, can lead to social isolation and the mental health issues associated with it, such as loneliness and depression.

THE SCENT OF SOMETHING NEW
Build your olfactory memory with unfamiliar smells

This week, try "learning" new scents.

Find new or unusual spices, herbs, or oils that are unfamiliar to you. Teach yourself to identify them by smell alone (no peeking!). Exercising your sense of smell will build your olfactory memory, and perhaps even boost the volume of your olfactory bulb, where scent memory resides.

➤ **WANT TO TAKE THIS TIP A BIT FURTHER?**
Certain aromas have been associated with health benefits. Try rosemary to enhance learning, lavender for calming and sleep, or citrus scents such as tangerine or orange for increased attention or energy.

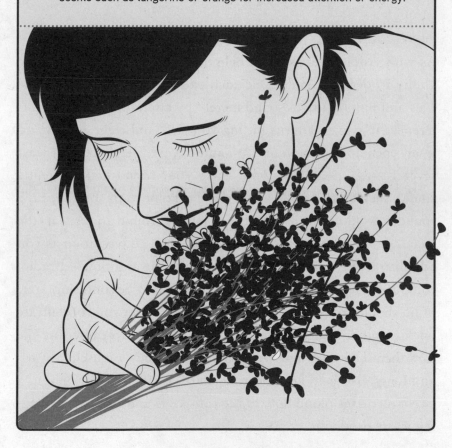

Most people experience some degree of presbycusis, or age-related hearing loss, and significant impairment strikes about a third of people older than 65. Loss of sharpness in the sense of hearing begins to be noticeable around age 50. Two common causes are changes in the auditory nerves and the buildup of wax in the ear canal. The latter can easily be remedied by a doctor's cleaning.

Age-related hearing loss can be slowed by practicing healthy habits. Any exercise that increases blood flow raises the level of life-giving oxygen available to the tissues surrounding the hair cells of the cochlea, likely extending their lives.

Have You Heard? Exercise Is the Secret

As with vision, exercises can help maintain or even increase the ability to detect sounds. One such exercise involves closing the eyes and pinpointing a sound merely by analyzing the slight differences in wave patterns hitting your left and right ears. Stand in an open area, shut your eyes, and have a friend stand at least several yards away from you. Have your friend make a gentle sound, such as clicking a metal cricket. Point to the origin of the sound. Keep pointing as your friend moves around and repeats the sound. In another exercise, try carrying on a conversation as you add distracting noises in the background one at a time—a radio, computer, television, and so on. Although it may be confusing, your brain should sort out the screening noises and let you concentrate on the sounds you want to follow. In addition to exercising the ears themselves, regular workouts of the body's muscles, heart, and lungs also help keep hearing sharp. Regularly working up a sweat increases blood flow to the ears' cells and removes damaging waste products.

▶ FLAVOR OF THE WEEK
How taste, smell, and touch evolve

The perceptions of taste, smell, and touch also change with time. The brain senses flavor through nerves embedded in taste buds that cover the tongue, as well as through specialized receptors in the nose. The senses of taste and smell grow weaker with age, as thresholds change. After age 60 or so, the ability to taste begins to wane for most, but not all, people, and the sense of smell declines as well. Salty and sweet tastes usually go first, followed by bitter and sour. The loss is gradual. In general, it takes a greater concentration of sweetness to taste something sweet, and a less intense sourness to taste something sour. Why this happens remains a bit of a mystery, but speculation centers on the fact that the mouth grows drier as saliva production decreases with age; environmental factors, too, add up over a lifetime. The number of taste buds also decreases with age, starting at about age 40 in women and age 50 in men. The remaining taste buds lose some of their mass, further reducing the surface area of the mouth sensitive to flavor. Other causes of diminished taste include tooth decay, mouth sores, certain medicines, and poor nutrition.

The Value of Sensitivity
The sense of touch also dulls a bit with age, typically lifting the threshold of sensation for pain, heat, cold, pressure, and vibration. Lowered sensitivity to heat and cold can be life-threatening, so it is recommended that the elderly cap their water heaters' maximum temperature at a safe level, and be careful to dress appropriately when they leave the house during periods of high heat and cold.

The origin of changes in skin receptors may be a reduction in blood flow, typically resulting from a more sedentary lifestyle and greater use of medications. Or it could be the aging process itself or health disorders that elderly people more commonly experience. One compensation occurs around age 70: As the skin grows thinner, it often becomes more sensitive to a light touch, such as the caress of a hand.

▶ NEW SENSATIONS
Fresh experiences enhance your senses

Challenging the senses in novel ways helps the brain keep existing neural pathways open and create new ones, allowing the brain to maintain and even expand its processing of information from the five senses. Leonard Katz, a neurobiologist, promotes the concept of exercising the brain by making multisensory associations. He says this can be done in two ways: by combining two or more senses in unexpected ways, or by using one of the five senses in a new context. The former might be appreciating a particular bit of music while smelling a pleasant aroma. Vivaldi's *Four Seasons,* seasoned with vanilla, for example. The latter technique might involve reliance on sound, touch, or sight to carry out a task that normally relies on the use of one sense. So, for example, your family might prepare and eat dinner in silence, using only visual cues to get everything set up, and then pass and use things on the table as needed.

Alternative Senses Kick In

You might also pretend to have lost your sense of sight for a short time. After you park the car in the garage, close your eyes, open the car door, and try to get into the house and hang up your coat. This might involve paying extra attention to the contours of your keys in order to pick out the right one for the door from the garage to the living room. Once you've found it and turned the lock, you would rely on touch and sound—the softness of the carpet under your feet after the tile of the entryway, the ticking of the mantel clock as an aural anchor to orient you as you make your way across the living

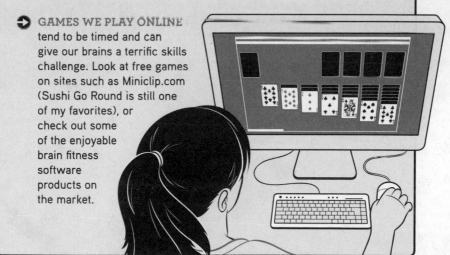

PLAY ONLINE
Now you have a good reason to spend time on online games

BRAIN BOOSTER

How would you like the chance to boost your brain power by taking ten minutes a day to play? What could be more fun than that?

➡ **RESEARCH HAS SHOWN** that we can better maintain intellectual skills, such as attention, speed, executive control, and memory (all of which can change as we age) by giving them a good workout. One of the best ways to keep these skills challenged is by playing games against the clock, since timed activities force us to focus, think fast, and be nimble in our approach.

➡ **GAMES WE PLAY ONLINE** tend to be timed and can give our brains a terrific skills challenge. Look at free games on sites such as Miniclip.com (Sushi Go Round is still one of my favorites), or check out some of the enjoyable brain fitness software products on the market.

WHAT'S IN THE BOX?

Your sense of touch needs exercise, too

Have you ever groped around your night table in the dark searching for your glasses or bottle of water? I bet you never considered while doing it that you were giving your tactile perception a workout.

Although we use our sense of touch constantly, rarely do we isolate the experience so that we focus solely on it. Even less likely are we to deliberately exercise that sense. Yet our tactile ability, like other aspects of our brain health, certainly can benefit from a workout.

Try this fun exercise to hone your sense of touch:

STEP 1
Take several small household objects (utensils, coins, paper clips, keys, small game pieces, and so on).

STEP 2
Place the objects together in a shoebox or similar size container.

STEP 3
Cover the box with a dish towel or other cloth.

STEP 4
Place your hand in the box under the cloth and try picking up the different objects and naming them using your sense of touch alone. How many can you identify correctly?

Want to take it up a notch? Try doing this exercise with your non-dominant hand.

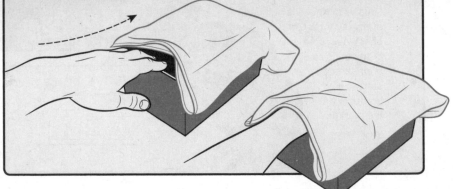

room—to complete your task. If you try this, go slowly, and try to re-create your house visually in your mind's eye. You'll find landmarks by touch and sound. Just don't storm ahead and bark a shin on the coffee table, or you'll get an unwanted sensory stimulation: pain.

Katz also recommends giving your senses a break from their routines. This can be as simple as taking a new route to work or rearranging the furniture in your living room.

BRAIN INSIGHT

Seeing With Your Tongue?

An experimental device can train other body parts to take the place of the eye

A scientist rolls a ball toward a woman in a chair. She reaches out her hand and stops it.

Nothing remarkable there, except the woman is blind. And she "saw" the ball with her tongue.

The blind woman's tongue was wired to a device called a BrainPort, itself wired to a video camera capturing the movements of the scientist and ball. BrainPort, originally developed by the late Paul Bach y Rita of Wicab Inc., works by substituting electrical impulses for other sensory stimuli. In this case, it trades the visual system's processing of light for encoded bursts of electricity sent to the brain through the surface of the tongue. (The tongue's sensitivity makes it ideal for maximum data communication.) The brain teaches itself how to interpret tongue-borne electrical bursts as if they had been delivered through the eyes. Similar research is under way to substitute or augment sensory information lost in the skin and ears, as well as compensate for a loss of balance. The vision centers of BrainPort users become active when processing electrical impulses from the skin.

Blind BrainPort operators, once trained, perceive size, shape, depth, and other visual qualities. Letters of the alphabet become clear.

Wicab is working toward release of a commercial version of the product.

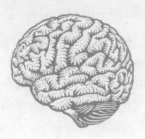

CHAPTER 4

A Body in Motion
How your brain keeps you moving steadily

For most people, grasping a pen from an outstretched hand, walking up a flight of stairs, or riding a bicycle seems a simple task. At one point, though, these skills required tremendous mental effort. It takes a baby months to learn to coordinate muscles, joints, and the sense of balance first to crawl, and then to master the antigravity circus of walking upright. During those early months, figuring out how to keep the body balanced, both at rest and in motion, requires fierce attention. Even so, the child toddles and falls a lot before learning the basics of walking.

Time passes, but still, the most basic of body movements arise from the brain directing an amazing, complicated symphony of three basic functions: movement of individual muscle fibers, coordination of muscle groups, and balance.

▶ FLEX, BEND, STRETCH
For every muscle movement, the mind is hard at work

....

Muscles move in response to the brain's conscious and unconscious orders, executed along nerve fibers. Electrochemical signals cause muscle fibers to contract. Even when you extend an arm or a leg, the process works only when the fibers contract—nerve signals never cause a muscle to stretch itself. These contractions act like binary digits: Muscle fibers either contract completely, 100 percent, or not at all. When your body needs extra strength, for lifting something heavy or twisting a stubborn jar lid, the brain recruits more and more muscle fibers to add their contractions to the existing total and increase the force your body applies.

Muscular Teamwork

Muscles work in groups. Shooting a basketball, for example, calls upon the brain to orchestrate the muscles of the fingers, hands, wrists, arms, shoulders, legs, thighs (bend your knees on those free throws!), and so on. The result, at least for a professional basketball player, is a smooth, well-coordinated movement that flows in properly executed order through muscles and joints to direct the basketball through the hoop. Without the brain's coordination of the sequence of neural firing, the ball might miss the rim, or even the backboard.

The brain could not pull off this amazing feat without a well-developed sense of balance. It's the body's response to gravity that keeps it upright. Without stable posture, muscle fiber contractions to reposition the body would have no foundation, no reference point. A dizzy or wobbly basketball player would never lead the league in scoring.

▶ MOTION CIRCUITS
Your brain as base command

Just how the brain coordinates movement became better understood in the late 19th century when British neurologist John Hughlings Jackson examined patients with epilepsy. He noticed that, in some patients, the convulsive movements associated with epilepsy seemed to flow in sequence from one body part to another. He concluded that muscular tics and jerks arose from the disorder affecting first one brain region and then another. The obvious conclusion was that discrete brain regions control movements in particular body parts.

Today, we know that most of the brain's circuitry is involved in both voluntary and involuntary movements. Key components include huge portions of the cerebrum, which houses the motor (movement) cortex; cerebellum; basal ganglia; brain stem; and the spinal cord, which not only carries signals to and from the brain but also organizes and responds to a variety of signals from the body's periphery. Most, if not all, of these parts of the nervous system work together to create movement. Movement is seldom the result of a single muscle's activation. Touching your nose with your forefinger activates muscles in your fingers, hand, arm, and shoulder, as well as your eyes. Executing the same motion while dizzy may call on other muscles to compensate.

Standing Tall

The spinal cord contains about 20 million axons. These nerve fibers, as well as those in the brain stem, neck, and legs, respond to gravity to keep the body stable and upright. Neurons in the brain stem and cerebellum react to slight changes in body position to automatically

TAP A TUNE

Let your fingers do the dancing while you're stuck at your desk

This Brain Booster is sure to get you moving to a different beat. Go ahead and make up a little tune by tapping your fingers on your table or desktop (the actual desktop, not the computer, though I guess you could make up a tune bopping on your computer if you are so inclined). You can use two hands or a nearby pen, if you like.

➤ CHOOSE YOUR OWN RHYTHM

Your tune can be short or long, simple or complex, though I would suggest going for more than just one "note." Tapping a tune will challenge your brain to think about the world in a slightly different way, and get you to coordinate your movement, auditory, and memory skills. Imagine—all that in just a few minutes today.

Who knows, you could even come up with your own personal theme song!

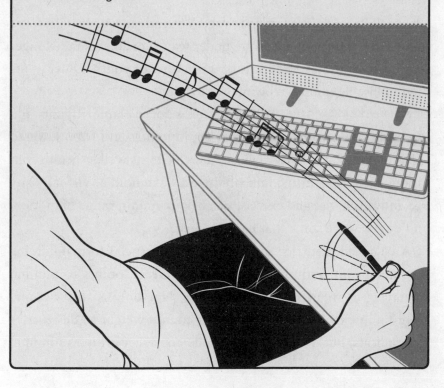

contract the right muscles in the right amount at the right time to maintain an upright posture. Damage to neurons in the cerebellum often announces itself by affecting the ability to stand upright for any length of time. Long-term abuse of alcohol can manifest itself in the cerebellum, resulting in an unsteady gait—or worse. Likewise, damage to crucial neurons from Parkinson's or stroke may impede movement in a variety of ways, from muscle rigidity to lack of balance. Certain health conditions, medications, and inner ear problems also affect the body's ability to maintain balance.

▶ HOW LOW CAN YOU GO?
Tracking flexibility through the years

Motor skills tend to degrade with age. With advancing years, it takes more time to get moving. Once under way, movements take longer to execute, and they lose some of the fluidity of youth. Older joints tend to lose flexibility, growing more rigid.

Science has discovered that age itself is not to blame. Rigidity and loss of flexibility, or range of motion, in joints stem from lowered levels of physical activity associated with age, as well as health conditions such as arthritis. Inflexibility can take hold at virtually any age. However, diet and exercise can help maintain range of motion, and even restore some that has been lost.

A balanced diet, rich in antioxidants, is crucial to maintaining maximum joint movement. Growing evidence points to vitamin C playing a singularly important role. Not only is this vitamin, plentiful in citrus fruits, an excellent counterweight to destructive free radicals, but it also helps the body construct proteins found in joint cartilage.

STRETCH AT YOUR DESK
Get rid of those deskbound doldrums

Spending all day at your desk or on the phone can really take a toll on your body and your mind. Taking small breaks to move, even in little ways, can help break the routine and give you a mental change of scenery.

➲ WIDE ARMS
Find a few minutes several times over the course of the day to get up from your desk and stretch. Try standing up and spreading your feet comfortably, to give yourself a firm base. Next, stretch your arms wide at shoulder's height. Then imagine a sense of pulling out toward your hands and feet to give yourself a nice stretch.

➲ BACKBEND
You can also try countering that hunched-over position we can find ourselves in at our desks by doing a gentle, slight backbend from your waist, or bending forward from the waist while seated in your chair and letting your arms and head dangle for a few moments (just be careful to protect your neck as you sit back up).

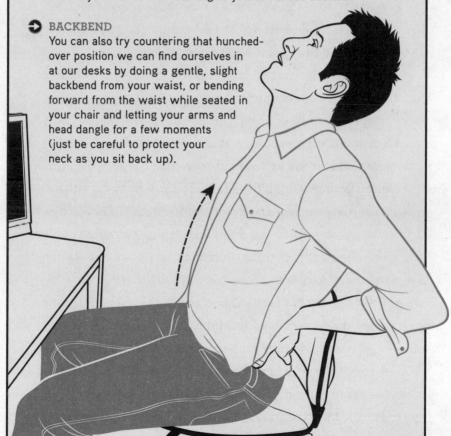

Keep That Spring in Your Step

Good exercises to maintain flexibility include stretches, which can be incorporated into a regular workout routine or performed by themselves. Stretching also has the added benefits of helping prevent injuries caused by muscle tightness and of reducing stress.

Tai chi, yoga, and Pilates classes can increase flexibility as well as balance. If you don't want to commit to a regimen of classes with a group, you can do some simple stretching exercises at home. Try these:

- ▶ **Warm-ups.** Cold stretches can cause muscle injuries. The best time to stretch is when muscles have already done some basic work and begun to heat up with energy and blood. So start with five to ten minutes of walking, pedaling on a stationary bike, or doing some other simple exercise.
- ▶ **Spine stretches.** Lie on your back on the floor with your arms and hands at your sides. With your legs straight, bring your feet up in the air. Try to raise them far enough to angle your feet back over your head. Count to five, lower your legs to the floor, and repeat ten times. This stretches your spine, an excellent way to minimize the risk of back injury.
- ▶ **Seated stretches.** Sit on the floor with your legs crossed and your back straight. Lean forward until your back is arched and your head and neck are parallel with the floor. Count to ten, then revert to your starting position. Repeat five times. When you're done, stand and get loose.
- ▶ **Trunk twists.** Stand with your hands on hips and arms akimbo. Your feet should be a short distance apart and

not move during the exercise. Twist your trunk slowly to one side and look behind you. Hold that position for five seconds. Then twist the other way and repeat. Do this a few times to stretch your trunk.

► **Leg lifts.** Stand next to a desk or table, positioned to one side of you. Grasp the edge with one hand. Slowly raise one leg until it is parallel to the floor. Lower the leg and repeat with the other leg. Do this ten times with each leg to boost flexibility in the hips.

If those exercises are too strenuous, you might try the following easier ones. Try repeating these three to six times at first, and then add more repetitions or go on to some of the previous exercises:

► **Reach for the sky.** Sit or stand so your back is straight. Raise your arms above your head and stretch for the ceiling. Return your arms to your sides to relax for a moment.

► **Side to side.** Stand tall with your feet apart and your arms at your sides. Bend to one side, letting your hand drag along your thigh toward your knee. Then straighten up. Bend to the other side, and repeat equally on both sides.

► **Toe loops.** While sitting in a chair, keep one leg bent while straightening the other before you. Stretch your toes toward your head and then downward. Then slowly circle the foot at the ankle. Repeat with the other foot.

► **Leg extensions.** Sit in a chair with your knees bent a bit. Straighten and stretch one leg before you, then let it drop. Repeat with the other leg.

▶ **Elbow loops.** Sit or stand with your elbows bent and your fingertips on your shoulders. Slowly rotate one of your elbows in a big, backward circle. Repeat with the other elbow. Or try simply bending and straightening the elbow again and again, which helps build arm flexibility.

▶ **Waist watchers.** Lean slightly forward while sitting in a chair with your knees bent and your feet on the floor. Bend forward slowly from the waist and stretch your hands toward your feet. Then slowly straighten and relax. After you've tried this exercise for a while, switch to a trunk twist. Put your right elbow on your left knee by twisting at the waist. Then straighten up, pause, and shift your left elbow to your right knee.

Be sure to breathe regularly, without holding your breath at any point. Don't bounce as you stretch, as bouncing tightens muscles and can cause minute scarring in muscle tissue. If you find any unpleasant level of discomfort from any of the exercises, stop immediately and try again another day. Persistent pain caused by simple exercises can be a sign you should see your doctor.

A Productive Form of Playtime

In addition to the previous exercises, you can invent your own or make use of your surroundings to promote strong balance

Tennis star Martina Navratilova, now in her mid-50s, likes to stretch with a foam roller, the kind sold in a sporting goods store. The roller stretches the fascia, connective tissues that surround the muscles, and improves blood flow, she told AARP.

TAKE A YOGA BREAK

How about bringing a little "om" into your life?

In many ways, yoga is the perfect brain health exercise. As a physical activity, yoga supports your more vigorous aerobic workouts by building strength and stamina (not to dismiss the fact that yoga itself can be aerobic, depending on your practice). In addition, yoga helps build sustained focus, which we all need to learn and remember on a daily basis. Finally, yoga is a terrific resource for maintaining emotional balance, and can be used to reduce stress, anxiety, and relieve depressed moods, all of which may lower our everyday mental performance.

➲ ACTIVITIES

Try taking a five-minute yoga break each day. Kripalu, a center for yoga in Massachusetts, offers a series of such breaks you can download to your computer or other media player (*www.kripalu .org*). If you have time and are feeling even more ambitious, try an online yoga class from Yoga Today (*www.yogatoday.com*) or another online source. Consider looking for yoga classes in your area and making yoga part of your path to better brain health.

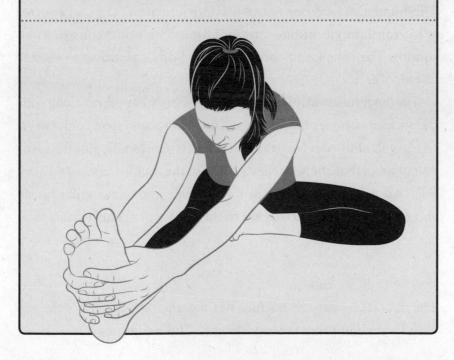

Stephen Jepson, in his early 70s, has converted his yard into a playground to keep his body and brain sharp. Jepson, featured in a video in the Growing Bolder Media Group's series celebrating active senior citizens, believes the key to staying mentally fit is to return to the playgrounds of childhood. Jepson challenges the movement-coordinating circuits of his brain by riding an elliptical bicycle, walking slack ropes strung between trees, hopping barefoot from rock to rock, and otherwise providing new and unusual stimulation to his motor cortex. The practice not only has maintained his balance and agility, he said, but has also sharpened his memory.

▶ IT ISN'T EASY BEING UPRIGHT
Your ears bear the burden of balance

The human ear carries out two important jobs. One, of course, is to translate vibrations into sensations the brain constructs as sounds. The other is to coordinate the body's position to keep it in balance.

The latter function relies on the vestibular system, which along with the cochlea occupies the inner ear. The vestibular system comprises a series of fluid-filled tubes called the semicircular canals, plus the vestibule, a space that connects the canals with the cochlea. Special sensory cells that detect motion occupy the vestibule and semicircular canals and send signals via nerve fibers to the pons and medulla oblongata.

Your Place in Space
The neural circuitry of balance ties together sensations in the ear with vision and other sensory systems. The brain uses the eyes and

specialized sensory cells in the feet to gather information about the position of the body in space. The vestibular system's fluid-filled tubes detect motion of the head, both in a straight line and in a curve. Fluid movement bends sensory neurons in the tubes, initiating electrical signals in the connecting nerve fibers. The brain swiftly integrates this incoming information and sends signals to the arms, legs, trunk, and other body parts to shift in reaction to changes in body orientation to the ground. The brain also directs the movement of the eyes to redirect their gaze, when necessary, to provide feedback as the body moves. So, for example, when you stumble, your eyes flash to the ground before you.

Proprioception is the brain's unconscious sense of the body's motion and spatial orientation. The system is amazingly complex and interconnected, yet you probably never give your balance a second thought—until you start to fall.

An Evolutionary Edge?

Anthropologists have noted an interesting fact about the vestibular system. Humans evolved over millions of years to walk upright on ground. This development freed the hands for carrying tools, such as axes, clubs, and spears that could aid in the hunt for food. Differences in the ability to coordinate upright movement may account in part for the extinction of humanity's evolutionary cousins, the Neanderthals. *Homo neanderthalensis* shared space with *Homo sapiens* until the former disappeared about 30,000 years ago. Recent examinations of Neanderthal skulls revealed that, compared with modern humans, Neanderthals had smaller vestibular systems. They would likely have had a less developed sense of balance and less agility. That could have made Neanderthal

GET JUGGLING

Keep those balls in the air and build some brainpower

Have you ever tried juggling? And not just your schedule?

➡ **WHY JUGGLE?**
Complex motor integration activities such as juggling have been shown to increase brain volume and improve everyday memory performance. Researchers in Germany found that juggling increased volume in the white matter of their subjects' brains. Such activities boost brain health by getting us to move and forcing us to focus and think about what we are doing. Best of all, they rate very high on the fun factor.

Chances are you may have tried juggling at one time in your life, only to give it up as too difficult. This is your chance to give juggling another shot. Start with one or two balls or scarves (scarves may be a bit easier at first) then slowly work your way up to three.

Want more direction? You can easily find instructional help on the Internet.

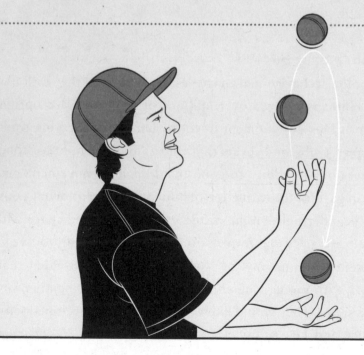

second best at hunting game, an evolutionary disadvantage in the long term.

As previously noted, aging causes the structure of the ear to change. Most notably, the eardrum thickens, which not only may affect hearing, but also impacts balance.

Staying Centered

Maintaining balance into old age is a key component of enjoying life. Journalist Scott McCredie, who wrote a book about the human sense of balance, said it's vital to challenge the sense of balance to keep it sharp. "[As] we move into our 60s . . . we can't afford not to think about it," he wrote. "Not just to prevent a potentially lethal fall, but to be able to continue moving gracefully through the world, to stay glued to the tightwire of life."

Two body systems linked to balance—vision, and the sensitivity of cells in the feet that inform the brain about the body's position— also typically decline with age. In addition, loss of muscle mass and less flexibility in the limbs mean that when an aging body begins to totter, the brain must rely on weakened tools to avoid a fall. Each year, one in three Americans older than age 65 loses balance and suffers a fall. Brittleness in elderly bones often causes them to break in such falls, sometimes with catastrophic results.

The sense of balance has two forms: static and dynamic. The former keeps the body upright when still. The latter maintains balance while the body changes its relationship with the surface of the Earth, as when climbing a hill or stairs, or turning a street corner on a bicycle. Both begin to gradually erode beginning in the body's third decade. Unless the deterioration is checked by deliberate steps, the result often is dizziness or loss of balance later in life. Compromised

balance may not seem like much of an impediment, but it can interfere with driving, walking, and even sitting upright. People with
continuing troubles with balance often have trouble holding a job.

▶ EASY DOES IT
Recognizing dizziness before a fall

Chronic dizziness increases the odds of falling by two to three times.
Dizziness is classified in four types, all of which become more common with advancing age:

- **Loss of balance;** unsteadiness; a feeling of being about
  to fall despite normal muscle strength. Disorders in the
  inner ear and the cerebellum, such as damage caused by
  alcoholism or stroke, can bring on this condition. So too
  can the use of too much sedative or anticonvulsant medication, as well as nerve disorders that affect the sensation
  of the position of the legs.
- **Faintness.** This feeling of impending blackout can stem
  from dehydration, nervous system disorders, abnormal heartbeat, and adverse reactions to blood pressure medication.
- **Vertigo.** This feels like movement in the body or the
  body's surroundings, despite both being at rest. Causes
  can include middle-ear infections, migraines, decreased
  blood flow to the brain, motion sickness, or something as
  simple and transitory as a sudden movement of the head.
- **Lightheadedness.** This vague feeling may arise from
  a panic attack, hyperventilation, depression, or other
  mental disorders.

WALK ON BACK

Put it in reverse and learn to walk all over again

Looking for a simple way to mix things up and challenge your coordination? Try walking backward.

➲ A NEW DIRECTION

Walking is something we do every day. In fact, it is one of our most overlearned motor activities (and one that gets parents most excited when their children first master it). So why not get your brain to focus differently by changing up this very simple, everyday activity?

Before you begin your backward walking, make sure that the area in which you are practicing is free of obstacles and has an even surface. Start slowly and walk carefully.

As you practice your "walk on back," notice how your sense of balance and coordination shifts. Chances are that the exercise will feel odd and awkward at first. But, like a child learning her first steps, you should find it gets easier the more you practice.

Exercises can maintain and even improve balance. Such exercises work the hips, knees, ankles, and feet. They also challenge the neurons of the vestibular system to keep it firing and wiring. These exercises require no special training: They're as easy as balancing on one foot for as long as you can, or walking by placing one heel directly in front of the toe of the other foot and continuing to walk in a straight line.

....

The Bird and the Snake
The peaceful benefits of a martial art

Legend says tai chi began when a 12th-century Taoist monk fled the cities to find peace in the mountains and wondered how to protect himself. The monk, Zhang Sanfeng (or Chang San-Feng), studied martial arts at his monastery, but an epiphany allowed him to move beyond his teachers. Zhang saw a bird and snake fighting. Instead of charging one another, the antagonists adjusted their movements to penetrate the adversary's defenses. Zhang saw that moving with an opponent's force, instead of opposing it, could be the foundation of a new martial art based on mimicking animals. Thus was born tai chi chuan, or "supreme ultimate fist."

Despite the martial name, tai chi today is practiced most often by those seeking inner peace instead of victory in combat. The dancelike, deliberate movements aim to bring mind, spirit, and body into alignment and operate them under a universal source of energy, called ch'i.

The discipline has a mystic, Eastern aura, but you don't have to understand how tai chi works to benefit from it. Its gentle, stress-free movements can be done at any age, but it has particular benefits for the elderly: Regular workouts improve balance, flexibility, and mobility, reducing the risk of falls. They may even combat depression.

....

Test Your Balance

Physical therapists Marilyn Moffat and Carole B. Lewis, authors of *Age-Defying Fitness,* suggest that before beginning a regimen to improve balance, you should assess your current state. They suggest the following exercises, to be performed near a table or some other sturdy piece of furniture you can lean on or grab as needed: Begin by putting on a pair of flat, closed shoes. Stand straight with your arms folded across your chest. Lift one leg until the knee is bent at about a 45-degree angle. Close your eyes and begin to time yourself; use a stopwatch if you have one. Stay balanced on one leg. Stop timing the exercise as soon as you uncross your arms, bend to one side more than 45 degrees, touch your bent leg to the floor, or move your foundation leg. When you're done, switch legs and start again.

Take your times and compare them to your age group. The norm for people 20 to 49 years old is 24 to 28 seconds. It drops to 21 seconds for people in their 50s, 10 seconds for those in their 60s, and 4 seconds for those in their 70s. Most people age 80 or older cannot count off even one second.

File away your numbers for comparison after dedicating yourself to the following exercise: Once again while wearing flat, closed shoes, stand near something you can grab. Plant your feet shoulder-width apart with arms stretched straight in front of you and parallel to the floor. Keep your eyes open. Lift one foot behind you by bending your knee about 45 degrees. Freeze for at least five seconds, if you can. Do this exercise five times, and then do exactly the same with the other leg. When you feel you have begun to make improvements, continue, but with your eyes closed.

You can practice this skill at any time during the day, such as when you're getting ready for work or bed. Incorporate a one-leg stand into brushing your teeth or combing your hair. (Best not to mix this exercise with a shaving razor, however.)

Sit and Stand

Another useful exercise boosts the strength of ankles, legs, and hips to help the body better deal with the potential dizziness of suddenly standing after sitting a long time. To get the most out of this exercise, sit up straight on something firm without having your back touch anything. Rise until you stand straight, and then sit again as quickly as you can without using your arms. Repeat three times at first. Over time, try to extend the exercise until you can do it ten times.

You also might specifically target the strength of your ankles by walking for a while on your toes, then switching to using only your heels.

BRAIN INSIGHT

More Than Monkeying Around

Neuroscientist Michael Merzenich at the University of California, San Francisco, has seen a brain physically change while learning a new task

Merzenich put a banana-flavored pellet in a cup and watched as a squirrel monkey extended an arm through the bars of a cage, grasped the pellet from the cup, and ate it. The test subject repeated the action dozens of times each day until it became automatic. Then Merzenich replaced the cup with a smaller one. It took a while for the monkey to fish the pellet out of the smaller cup, but it eventually mastered that skill, too. Twice more, Merzenich swapped the cup for a smaller one, until the monkey had become extremely adept at getting a banana pellet from a narrow opening by the fourth cup.

Computer images of the monkey's brain revealed that the neural networks associated with conscious finger manipulation expanded as the monkey learned greater dexterity. However, once a monkey no longer had to think about the motions, the expanded neural networks active during the learning phase showed reduced activity. The skill moved from the parts of the brain associated with conscious thought to other parts that handled routine movements.

The learning circuits of squirrel monkey brains, and those of humans, don't need to stay burdened with old information. To use a computer analogy, they can clear their memory after mastering a task to prepare themselves for a new one.

BRAIN INSIGHT ···

Technology Lends a Hand

Sensors implanted in the brain can command electronic limbs

It's not much of a stretch to go from manipulating a computer cursor with a thought, accomplished in 1998 and depicted a few years later on the television drama *House M.D.*, to moving something more substantial. In May 2012, a team of scientists announced that they had taught two quadriplegics to manipulate a robotic arm. The arm reached and grabbed, just like one of flesh and blood. One of the two people, a woman who had been unable to give herself a drink for 15 years, smiled broadly when she wrapped robotic fingers around a coffee cup and took a sip.

The arm receives electrical impulses from an aspirin-size sensor implanted in the motor cortex. When the test subjects imagine making particular arm movements, the sensor picks up patterns of neural firing, translates them into signals that can be read by the arm, sends them along a wire, and sets the arm in motion.

The arm rests on a shoulder-height dolly and has yet to leave the lab. Researchers at Brown University, the Department of Veterans Affairs, and the German Institute of Robotics and Mechatronics hope to develop a wireless transmission system as well as lifelike limbs that are integrated into the body.

··

Tai Chi

Tai chi, an ancient Chinese muscle-training discipline, appears to be one of the most effective systems of improving balance. Studies have shown practitioners of its slow, deliberate movements decrease their likelihood of falling. Tai chi is not only a discipline of exercise, it's also a form of meditation; Chinese practitioners call it "mindful exercise." Studies at the University of Massachusetts Medical School at Worcester reveal that the combination of physical and mental exercises in tai chi can lower anger, depression, and tension.

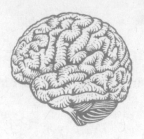

CHAPTER 5

Name That Tune

When words get stuck on the tip of your tongue

At the ancient Greek town of Delphi, an oracle—a woman chosen for her purity—sat atop a tripod next to a hole in the ground. According to legend, the god Apollo had earlier tossed the body of the monstrous serpent Python into that very opening. Gases from the decomposing body rose to the surface and met the nose of the Delphic oracle. She inhaled and fell into a trance in which Apollo spoke to her. The oracle shared her revelations, prophesying to the people. But she did so in an unintelligible tongue. Thus, the oracle at Delphi knew great truths, but could not communicate them in plain language. Priests of the temple came to her rescue, translating the oracle's gibberish for the people.

A modern-day, medical parallel to the oracle's problem can be found in a rare disease called Wernicke's aphasia. It strikes the nerve fibers in a particular part of the posterior temporal lobe. People with this disorder lose their ability to understand language and speak intelligibly. Their words often come out with apparently good syntax, but they make no sense. A so-called "word salad" of a patient with Wernicke's aphasia might sound like this: "Fly to the oven and get the government mystery. Repeat the library, fourteen alphabet monster."

▶ WHAT'S THAT WORD AGAIN?
When you know what to say but just can't say it

The conditions of the oracle and a patient with Wernicke's aphasia lie at the extreme end of a scale of language-processing difficulties. At the lower end lies the occasional problem of searching for, but not finding, the right word to say. Somewhere between the two is the paradox of the aging brain's skill with language. If a brain stays active and builds vocabulary, it may have a far richer treasure trove of words from which to choose than a much younger brain. But an aging brain struggles more to find the words it wants. Wise elders sometimes wrestle with the maddening problem of knowing what they want to say, but being unable to retrieve the correct words from memory—and the problem typically increases with age.

Scientists call this problem the "tip of the tongue" experience, which occurs when a word exists in a person's lexicon but temporarily remains inaccessible to the brain. It's a normal part of aging—tip-of-the-tongue problems typically begin around age 40—and is reported as one of the most frequent and troubling problems of older adults. As brains mature into middle age and beyond, they think more deliberately, and for a longer time, before making decisions. They may know the answer to a question, but fail to come up with it quickly.

SENTENCE SCRAMBLE
Make sense of nonsense and exercise your brain

Word games can be addictive. Many of us love these puzzles, and they are without doubt the most popular kind of brain game among adults.

How are word games good for our brains? Such activities grab our attention, get us to make new connections, and give us the chance to "stretch" our minds and think outside of our mental box.

Here's a word game you may not have played before—Sentence Scramble. It's a quick diversion that gives your creativity a boost as well. To play:

➡ STEP 1
Find a newspaper, magazine, or book and turn to a random page.

➡ STEP 2
Select a paragraph (any one will do) and go through it. Write down every fifth word, until you have a list of eight to ten words.

➡ STEP 3
Now you are ready to play! Take that list and make up a sentence, using only those words—the quirkier and sillier your sentence, the better.

SAUCER	FENCE	RADIO
POSTER	ROCK	GIRAFFE
CALENDAR	JUMP ROPE	BUMPER

Research associate Meredith Shafto of Britain's University of Cambridge studies normal cognitive aging. She told the *Washington Post* that tip-of-the-tongue experiences are "part of what we call normal or healthy aging . . . With normal aging there are changes that are noticeable and distressing and irritating, but they are not pathological."

▶ WHERE IT ALL HAPPENS
The insula, word choice central in your brain

A research team led by the Pomona College Project on Cognition and Aging, and headed by Deborah Burke, discovered that tip-of-the-tongue experiences increase as the density of neurons in a brain region called the left insula decreases. The insula, deep between the frontal and temporal lobes, recently has drawn neurologists' attention for a variety of reasons. It has been linked to neural processing of sound. It lights up in brain scans when the body feels or anticipates pain, empathizes with others, desires a drug, or responds to jokes or music.

Use Them or Lose Them

Burke's team relates the insula's age-related decline in gray matter to a theory equating atrophy with disuse: Neural connections that encode words grow weak and decline if those words aren't often spoken aloud. Those neural connections are scattered around the brain, but the insula may be a key performer in the networks' reconstruction of words.

"We like to think of words as being stored in a unit in our head, and that we have a little place in our minds where we have [for example] Brad Pitt, and we know what he looks like and what movies he's been in and his name and all that," she told the *Washington Post*. But word-related information isn't stored in such an integrated way. Various neural circuits encode how a word sounds, what it means, how it fits into the syntax of language, how it's associated with images, and so on. The brain can lose access to one part of the related circuits and not the others.

Polyglots

Verbal fluency reaches a peak in people who speak dozens of languages

Bilingual people speak two languages. Trilingual people speak three. Those fluent in four or more are polyglots, Greek for "many tongues."

The most famous polyglot in the United States was probably Thomas Jefferson. He fluently spoke and read English, Greek, Latin, French, Italian, and Spanish. Jefferson also attempted German and dabbled in Arabic, Gaelic, and Welsh.

Other notable polyglots included Heinrich Schliémann, excavator of the ancient city of Troy, who spoke German and at least 12 other languages, and Jean-François Champollion, who spoke more than a dozen languages by age 20, and went on to crack the puzzling hieroglyphs of the fabled Rosetta stone.

One of the most amazing polyglots was German diplomat Emil Krebs. By the time he entered Berlin's Foreign Office school for interpreters, he already spoke a dozen languages. He insisted on learning the toughest ones, which led him to Mandarin. In a few years, he was sent to China as Germany's chief interpreter. The empress dowager took tea with him to enjoy hearing him speak. By his death in 1930, Krebs had learned at least 65 languages, including Armenian, which he grasped in nine weeks. Postmortem examinations of his brain revealed unusual cellular organization in Broca's area, a region associated with speech.

Is a Rose a Rose?

The circuits for word sounds and objects appear to be particularly vulnerable to decay because there seldom is a logical connection, except for onomatopoeic words such as *bang* and *splat,* which take their names from their sounds. Why is a rose called a rose?

DO A WORD SEARCH
A familiar word game is great verbal exercise

This word search game gives your brain a boost by pressing you to be more nimble in your thinking and to shift your usual way of seeing things. Take the following words and see how many other words you can come up with, using only the letters of the original word.

➲ HAPPY SEARCHING!
Working the word is a simple activity, yet a great way to get a quick mental workout and intellectual challenge.

Want to up the ante? Give yourself one minute a word.

RESOLUTION	SYNAPSE
SUFFICIENT	PROPAGATION
BENEFICENCE	IMPRESSIVE

As a result of this disconnect between a word and the thing it represents, you might recognize Brad Pitt in a magazine photograph but not recall his name. Your brain's connection to the network containing his name deteriorates. This happens when the circuits lie dormant for too long, and leads to so-called "transmission deficits." If you don't hear the name Brad Pitt while looking at his face, the connection can wither.

Sounds are more vulnerable to decay than other kinds of experiences, Burke said. That would explain why you can know a word, and know you know it, but struggle with the tip-of-the-tongue experience to retrieve it.

NAME THAT CATEGORY
Reinforce your verbal recall with a name game

Here's a fun, short exercise that will build on your ability to think of words quickly (always a challenge as we grow older) and test your recall.

➲ ANIMALS, ANIMALS
Get a piece of paper and pen or pencil. Set a timer for two minutes (or just keep track on your watch or phone). Ready? Go ahead and write down as many animals as you can in those two minutes. They can be from the land or the sea, the jungle or the desert—just see how many you can come up with in that time frame.

➲ CHANGE CATEGORIES
You can keep this exercise going by simply changing categories each time. Try using foods, plants, colors, countries—anything you can categorize will work well. See if your lists become longer as you become more practiced at this exercise.

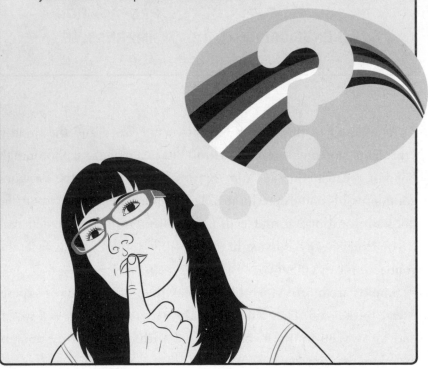

▶ PRIMING THE PUMP
Improving the flow from thinking to saying

Burke and other researchers discovered that the recall of tip-of-the-tongue words increased with "phonological priming." That's a fancy way of saying that when a person struggling to come up with a word on the tip of the tongue experiences other words containing similar sound—especially the initial sound, number of syllables, and stress patterns of the hidden word—the desired word often comes to mind. For example, aiming at the target word *Velcro,* Burke's team supplied to test subjects the words *venerable, pellet, decreed, overthrow,* and *mistletoe.* For the target word *Columbus,* Burke's team supplied the words *cologne, conniver, alumnus, omnibus,* and *amoebas.* Reading and saying aloud those words brought success. "It has been suggested that a [tip-of-the-tongue] target word pops into mind 'spontaneously' when phonological components of the word occur inadvertently during conversation," Burke's team wrote. Perhaps trying to think of words similar to the missing one will help, especially if the word's initial sound can be recalled. If you're stuck in a tip-of-the-tongue moment, Burke recommends focusing on words that spring into your mind as you search for the missing target. Their related sounds may prime the pump and restore connection to the lost word or phrase.

The Pomona College Project on Cognition and Aging's research on the insula and tip-of-the-tongue problems predicts that keeping neural connections strong for a broad vocabulary will reduce failures to find a particular word. "Using language in ordinary activities like socializing or in games like Scrabble may help keep words accessible and off the tip of the tongue," the project's team wrote. Reading aloud and talking to people at dinner may help maintain the neural circuits associated with words and sounds.

There isn't much you can do for retrieving names from your past, but you can increase the strength of encoding for current acquaintances. That's a memory-enhancing skill discussed in Chapter 7.

▶ FINDING THE RIGHT WORDS
Keeping your brain fluent

Tip-of-the-tongue problems form a subset of verbal fluency studies. Verbal fluency is the ability to quickly and smoothly access vocabulary when writing or speaking. It typically declines with age, and also can be affected by developmental disabilities, brain injuries, cancer, and some neurological disorders. It is not a strong measure of intelligence, as some smart people do poorly on verbal fluency tests.

Tests of verbal fluency sometimes are used as indicators of possible cognitive impairment, as they may reflect changes in the brain's word-processing centers. In a typical test, doctors might give a patient 60 seconds to list as many words as possible that start with the letter "P." The test taker counts and analyzes the words, as some might not fit the criteria. The 1996 movie *Phenomenon* depicts a verbal fluency test. In one scene, a doctor asks an ordinary man whose cognitive functions have been enhanced to name as many mammals as he can in 60 seconds. The test subject responds by instantly reeling off 26 mammals in alphabetical order from aardvark to zebra.

GET VERBAL
A word a day keeps the doctor away

Resources readily at hand on your shelf or via your computer can help get your mind engaged by expanding your vocabulary. Building your word skills can really make you think and is a great prep for word games, writing, and other intellectual challenges. Research has demonstrated that such mental activities may reduce our risk for serious memory impairment by as much as 26 percent. And this exercise is fast, free, and fun!

➲ **THERE ARE SOME GREAT ONLINE SOURCES** for getting more out of your vocabulary. Try Freerice.com (and donate rice to the World Food Programme at the same time), or sign up for one of several sites to receive a "Word of the Day." You can also simply pull out the dictionary—an old-fashioned approach to building your vocabulary that still works!

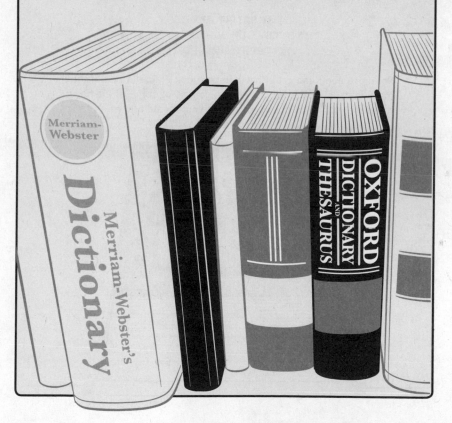

WRITE A HAIKU

This Japanese verse, which can be easily learned,
will stretch your word skills

· ·

What better way to boost your brainpower than with a mind-stretching exercise certain to be poetry to your ears? Writing haiku is a wonderful way to get out of your "boxed-in" brain and challenge yourself to think differently and creatively.

Haiku is a time-honored Japanese form of verse dating back centuries. Haiku is known for its simple form, which in its traditional English-language version requires a pattern of five syllables, seven syllables, and five syllables. Classical haiku also makes use of images that are seasonal and sensory in nature.

Although I am by no means a haiku expert, here's my try at this exercise to get you going:

> SHE SAT AT HER DESK
> THE SNOW GLISTENED IN THE SUN
> THE TREE SHIVERED COLD.

For more about the art of haiku, take a look online at one of the many instructional sites or find translations of some of the haiku masters, such as Basho or Buson, at your local library.

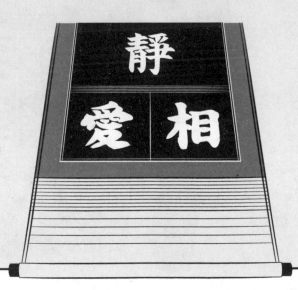

BRAIN INSIGHT

Learning To Speak Again

Congresswoman Gabrielle Giffords shows just how resilient the brain can be

I pledge allegiance . . . to the flag . . ." By leading the pledge at the 2012 Democratic National Convention, former Arizona Congresswoman Gabrielle "Gabby" Giffords demonstrated how far she had come. And how far she still has to go.

Giffords was shot through the left side of her brain in January 2011. Details of her injuries have never been made public. However, the left hemisphere controls speech and right-side body movement. Giffords suffered impaired mobility and aphasia, the inability to speak.

Music therapy helped her talk again. While the left side of the brain controls language, both hemispheres process music. In an amazing feat of neuroplasticity, Giffords' singing therapy helped her brain move her speech functions to the right hemisphere. She still slurred a few words and walked stiffly at the convention, but her achievement touched many viewers.

Traumatic brain injury can strike anyone. But you can do two things to reduce your risk. One is to protect your head with a helmet when riding a bike or motorcycle, or engaging in rough sports. The other is to build up your cognitive reserve to make your brain more richly connected and to increase its plasticity, should it ever be needed.

Talk, Talk, Talk

The subject of *Phenomenon* achieved greater verbal fluency via a terminal brain tumor that created new neural pathways. Not a pleasant option for cognitive enhancement, to say the least. More practical methods of improving verbal fluency, and cognitive strength in general, focus on general health. Sleep deprivation can decrease verbal fluency, as can a poor diet. Studies have shown that skipping breakfast, for example, can hurt verbal fluency, apparently by depriving the brain of its optimal nutritional needs. On the other hand, obesity has been linked to lowered verbal fluency and other cognitive functions. In particular, a 2010 study of more than 8,000 postmenopausal women using data from the Women's Health Initiative, a major national U.S. health study, found that as a person's body mass index rose, cognitive functions tended to decline. The group performing the worst on tests of verbal fluency and other cognitive tasks had a high ratio of hip circumference to waist size, meaning they carried excess weight on their hips.

If you want to improve your verbal fluency, try exposing your brain to new vocabulary words as well as new ways of putting them together. With practice, words become more familiar and you are more apt to easily retrieve them. If you read only the business section of the paper, you'll know plenty of business-related words, but you'll be less fluent in other lexicons. So try reading the editorial page or the sports section. If you're reading online or on a handheld digital device, you can easily look up unfamiliar words. If you go to the trouble of mastering new words by processing and understanding them in context, you'll strengthen verbal fluency.

World's First Word Processor

An individual's cognitive resources dramatically affect the ability to recall spoken and written words. As older adults usually have less working memory than their younger counterparts, it makes sense that they must make greater demands on their working memory to process language as they grow older. Studies in the 1990s demonstrated that older adults have good comprehension when they hear simple, short sentences spoken aloud because they don't tax the working memory as much as longer, more complex ones. But in controlled experiments, older adults showed more difficulty in language processing than younger adults as sentences sprouted more clauses and phrases. The difference appears both in accurate recall of the words themselves as well as comprehension of their meaning. Too much information, delivered too quickly, can overload an elderly brain.

On the other hand, the brains of older adults work with nearly youthful efficiency when processing communications such as spoken conversations and instructions that are delivered in short, simple bursts. The decline in processing of language is not as big a problem for text on a page for obvious reasons: If the reader misses something on the first pass, he or she can back up and reread the difficult passage—at a slower pace, if necessary.

Music to Your Ears

Memory for spoken words has been shown to be stronger in mature adults if they had musical training before the age of 12. A 1998 study at Chinese University in Hong Kong revealed that adults who learned how to play a musical instrument as a child scored 16 percent higher on tests for word memory than those who had no such training. The sample was small—a total of 60 college students—but the results nevertheless were intriguing. Thirty students who had at least six years of musical training before they turned 12 demonstrated better recall of words read aloud from a list than a group of 30 who lacked comparable musical training. The memory enhancement did not extend to visual designs, which usually are processed in the brain's right hemisphere. The musically trained students had no advantages at remembering and drawing simple designs they saw.

Neural plasticity apparently explains the Hong Kong study's results. Brain scans of professional musicians have noted an expanded region of neurons in the left planum temporale, a roughly triangular region of the temporal lobe. The region plays a role in processing not only music but also verbal memory. The research supports other work suggesting that musical training prepares the brain for more than just music. Learning to read and play music requires the brain to rapidly recognize and process groups of symbols. Enhanced sensitivity to grouping of symbols likely transfers to the symbols of letters, standing for sounds, that join to form words.

▶ PARLEZ-VOUS
The power of learning a second language

Decades ago, some scientists believed that learning a second language caused linguistic confusion or even cognitive deficits in young children. Instead, the brains of bilinguals, as children and adults, tend to have a stronger executive function than those of people who speak only one language. The executive function, centered in the prefrontal cortex, keeps the brain focused on what's important. It supports the ability to hold two things in the mind and switch back and forth as needed, such as conversing while following a game on television. Or it can tune out distractions to focus concentration. Children who learn a second language generally are better able than their one-language counterparts to maintain attention while being bombarded with irrelevant stimulation.

"If you have two languages and you use them regularly," cognitive neuroscientist Ellen Bialystok of York University in Toronto told the *New York Times*, "the way the brain's networks work is

LEARN A NEW LANGUAGE
Brain travel to foreign lands has its rewards

Learning a new language seems to be one of the most popular ways in which folks keep their brains sharp. Although mastering a new language can become more difficult as we grow older, the task itself is one that many of us seem to find compelling and engaging. Often, it is something we have wanted to do for many years, or it gives us a chance to perhaps recapture the language of our grandparents or great-grandparents. Without doubt, the process of learning a new language is a terrific challenge that can build new connections in the brain.

➲ FIGURE OUT WHICH LANGUAGE YOU'D LIKE TO STUDY. Next, look at the many resources for learning that new language and figure out which path you'd like to take. You can attend a class or take one online, find a tutor, or use a language program. Even better, why not plan a trip to the country that is home to your newly mastered tongue?

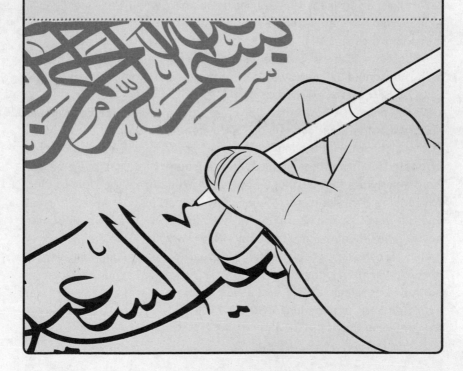

that every time you speak, both languages pop up and the executive control system has to sort through everything and attend to what's relevant in the moment. Therefore, the bilinguals use that system more, and it's that regular use that makes that system more efficient."

BRAIN INSIGHT

Telepathic Tweeting

Your thoughts in 140 characters or fewer

In early April 2009, University of Wisconsin biomedical doctoral student Adam Wilson prepared to send the first message that could be described as telepathic.

Wired magazine likened the event to the moment when Alexander Graham Bell, inventor of the telephone, sent his assistant what Bell said was the first phone message: "Mr. Watson, come here. I want to see you."

Wilson's message was more a simple announcement of what he was doing, and could be seen by anyone with access to the Internet: "USING EEG TO SEND TWEET."

Wilson manipulated a computer program that recognized changes in his brain activity patterns when he concentrated on particular letters of the alphabet. His thoughts moved a cursor and selected letters to be posted to his microblogging Twitter account. The interface emerged from a software tool developed by Justin Williams of the University of Wisconsin's Neural Interface Technology Research and Optimization Lab and Gerwin Schalk, a neural injury specialist at the Wadsworth Center, a public health laboratory in upstate New York.

Medical uses being explored for this program include opening avenues of communication with patients who have "locked-in" syndrome and cannot move or speak. Wilson's subsequent brain-to-computer messages indicated other applications. "GO BADGERS," tweeted the University of Wisconsin football fan.

A Word for Everything, and Every Word in its Place

That's important for success as teens and adults. Barbara Lust, a developmental psychology and linguistics expert at the Cornell Language Acquisition Lab, says a strong executive function is "responsible for selective and conscious cognitive processes to achieve goals in the face of distraction." Those goals include academic readiness and success, both as children and later as adults.

Enhanced cognition for bilinguals extends into old age. Bialystok found that bilingual elderly adults outperform monolinguals on tasks that test executive function. Furthermore, after studying the records of 400 patients with Alzheimer's, she found that bilingual people exhibited symptoms of the disease an average of five to six years later than monolingual people. These findings appear to support a study of the nuns of Mankato, Minnesota, that suggested correlations between higher levels of education early in life, as well as expanded cognitive reserves of an enriched brain, with maintenance of cognitive functions, sometimes despite physical evidence of the initial stages of Alzheimer's.

► START EARLY
Four-year-old translators do it with ease

Although humans can add a second language at any time, the best and easiest time to learn is early childhood. Young children who learn two languages at the same time don't have the adult disadvantage of their primary language interfering with their acquisition of new sounds, grammar, and meaning. "When you're a kid, all you're working at is acquiring a language, and you don't have anything to get in the way of that," Lisa Davidson, an associate professor of linguistics at New York University, told *Forbes*. "When you're an adult and you already have a language, the one you already know filters sounds and you get substantial interference from it."

Immersion of a child in an environment where two languages are spoken all the time smooths the path to bilingualism. Hearing multiple speakers controls against acquiring an accent that is particular to one person. The sooner a child learns a second language, the more likely the child will master the accents and tones of a native speaker.

Steps to a Second Language

The Cornell Language Acquisition Lab recommends the following to help a child learn a second language:

- ▶ **Surround the child** with conversations and social settings that expose him or her to the extra language.
- ▶ **If the child** is learning a second language outside the home, keep the heritage language of the child's family at home.
- ▶ **Give the child opportunities** to play with children who speak the second language.
- ▶ **Read** and tell stories in both languages.
- ▶ **Share music,** film, and other fun language-learning environments in both languages.

Young people and adults have different aptitudes for learning a nonnative language, just as they have aptitudes for math or geography. Experts agree that the best way to master a second language varies with the individual. But in general, learning a second language gets harder with age.

Find Your Path and Stick With It

To find their best learning method, adults might try audio or audio-visual programs, classes, conversations with native speakers, or immersion in the second language. When they find what works, they should stick with it. The key is to work a bit every day on acquiring the new language, and then expand vocabulary and sophistication. After achieving fluency, challenging the brain further might involve going to a higher level of instruction, such as taking a history or political science class in the second language. ◆

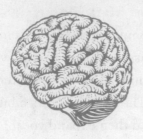

CHAPTER 6

Attention, Please

Focusing on what's in front of you

A music teacher who appeared to have unusual vision problems went to his ophthalmologist, but the doctor could not help him. He referred the man to neurologist Oliver Sacks, in hopes that a brain specialist could succeed where an eye specialist could not.

Sacks saw the man and his wife during an office visit. The man, whom Sacks calls "Dr. P.," acted strangely. He cocked his head to face Sacks with his ears, not his eyes. And when Dr. P. did turn his gaze toward Sacks, it flicked from place to place in an unnatural way. Sacks sensed that Dr. P. was checking out his features one at a time. When the visit was over, Dr. P. got ready to leave. He reached for his wife's head and tried to lift it as if it were his hat. His wife reacted as if it happened all the time.

For the next visit, Sacks went to Dr. P.'s home. Sacks wore a rose in his jacket lapel, but Dr. P. could not fathom what it was. He described it as "a convoluted red form with a green attachment." Only when Dr. P. smelled the rose did he realize what it was.

Like this subject, described in Sacks's book *The Man Who Mistook His Wife for a Hat,* a man in England also developed a strange change in his brain's visual processing system late in life. In 1988, the man, named John in the story related in *The Tell-Tale Brain* by Vilayanur S. Ramachandran, went into the hospital for an operation to remove his appendix. While there, the 60-year-old suffered a stroke that destroyed a part of his brain. When John's wife walked into his room, he no longer recognized her face. Nor could he recognize anyone's face, for that matter—not even his own. John told his doctor that he could see perfectly well. What he couldn't do was recognize objects instantly. Shown a carrot, John said, "It's a long thing with a tuft at the end—a paint brush?"

Missing the Big Picture

Both men had a form of visual agnosia, a disorder that keeps the brain from recognizing or understanding the visual signals it receives via the retinas. Patients with agnosia often can describe shape, color, texture, and other details of what they see but cannot put the whole picture together. Typically, the disorder arises from damage to the posterior occipital lobes, home of the visual cortex, and the temporal lobes. John's particular case included prosopagnosia, the inability to recognize faces. People with the condition often develop coping strategies, such as John's technique of recognizing his wife by her voice. Interestingly, Sacks discovered in middle age that he had some degree of prosopagnosia himself. He had great difficulty with faces, especially when seeing them out of context. He realized that, beginning as a child, he recognized people by individual characteristics—a pink dress, big eyebrows, a thatch of red hair, and so on.

SEE SQUARED

Sharpen your perceptions by spotting shapes in your surroundings

Puzzles that challenge your perception are a great way to give your visual abilities a good workout. Even the familiar childhood challenge of finding shapes in a complex setting can help adult perceptions.

➲ **LOOK AT THE PICTURE BELOW,** for instance. How many squares can you find?*

➲ **WANT TO STAY SQUARED?** Try looking for squares in your surroundings, such as in your office or family room. Challenge other family members, colleagues, or friends to find the squares with you and see who can find more.

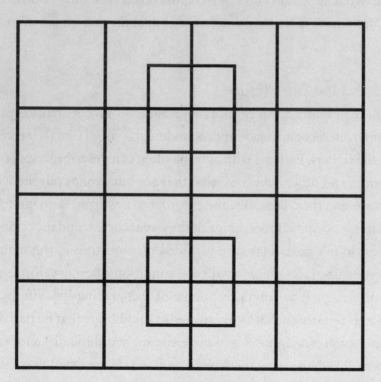

*Up to 40! Don't forget the 3x3 squares.

The Complex Mind's Eye

For the vast majority of children and adults, visual perception works easily and unconsciously. You look upon the world, and it makes sense. But that's because 30 visual areas of the cortex synchronize their work to process individual bits of visual data, provide feedback to one another, and assemble an image. Once light bounces off an object, enters the eye, and is focused on the retinas, it is broken into electrical impulses. These impulses—like dots and dashes of Morse code—fly to the visual cortex for sophisticated processing. It no longer makes sense to speak of whole "images" in the brain. Signals for shape, color, movement, and so on go through processing before the brain's visual networks construct a comprehensible representation of the world in the "mind's eye." Failure anywhere along the line can cause trouble. You can have fully functioning eyes and still not see.

► LOOK AGAIN
Illusions Test Visual Perception

The brain's role in constructing meaning out of what you see is easily demonstrated by optical illusions.

Illusions can emerge from retinal processing of the visual primary colors of red, green, and blue in the eye's cone cells, or deeper in the brain's neural networks. Two good examples of illusions resulting from neural processing are the Necker cube and Ames room. The former takes its name from the Swiss crystallographer Louis Albert Necker, who was looking at a cubic crystal through a microscope in 1832, when the back and front sides of the cube seemed to spontaneously flip. Necker repeated the illusion by devising a simple drawing of a transparent wire-frame cube whose perspective shifted as he gazed upon it. The viewer's brain imposes order on the cube by selecting one face to be the one closest to the eyes. However, in short order, the brain switches orientation, sending the previously foremost square face to the back side. The brain chooses one perspective or the other, and cannot hold both images in mind at the same time.

The Ames room, named for inventor Adelbert Ames, Jr., is a grossly distorted room of trapezoidal shape that, when viewed from one point directly front and center, appears to have normal right-angled walls, floor, and ceiling. One corner opposite the viewer is much farther away than the other, but clever manipulation of perspective makes the room seem rectangular with the far wall parallel to the room's front. A person in the far corner seems tiny while another person in the near corner appears gigantic; walking from one corner to the other makes a person appear to grow or shrink. The illusion works because the brain insists that the room must be a three-dimensional rectangular shape, which it has been conditioned to expect.

A Slam Dunk Advantage?

Illusions can have a practical side, tricking the brain into improving performance.

Psychologist Jessica Witt of Purdue University, who won a gold medal at the World Games as part of an Ultimate Frisbee team, examines the phenomenon of altered perception among athletes—those moments when the basketball rim seems larger or smaller, or the tennis net seems to get higher or lower. She noted that softball and tennis players report that when they're hitting well, their brains perceive the ball as larger than normal. Witt performed a study, published in 2012, to make a golf cup seem larger. She and co-authors Dennis R. Proffitt of the University of Virginia and Sally A. Linkenauger of the Max Planck

Institute-Tübingen set up a golf hole on a ramp. A projector shone 11 small circles around the cup, creating the illusion of the cup appearing larger than its normal diameter of four and one-quarter inches. College students using the optically enhanced cup sank 10 percent more putts than those without the enhancement. Expanding on her research, Witt said visual distractions confuse the brain and make it harder for athletes to perform. Crazy fans wagging giant foam fingers under the basket may actually alter the performance of free-throw shooters.

BRAIN INSIGHT

Finding Waldo

The search for the cartoon figure involves a coordinated mental effort

You probably know Waldo. Tall, thin. Wears jeans, a red-and-white pullover, and a matching cap. Round eyeglasses. Gets lost in crowds. For years, neuroscientists were split on how the brain orchestrated the search for Waldo's tiny cartoon image amid huge illustrations in the popular Where's Waldo? children's books of Martin Handford. Some said the brain's visual system worked like a spotlight, moving from image to image, in a manner known as serial processing. Others said the visual system took in the entire illustration and then used its focusing abilities to pull Waldo's colors and shapes out of the jumble, in a manner known as parallel processing.

Turns out, both sides had part of the answer, according to Robert Desimone, director of the McGovern Institute for Brain Research at MIT. He led a study tracking brain activity in macaque monkeys executing a Waldo-like search. His team found that neurons in the V4 region of the visual cortex synchronize their signals to direct attention toward colors and shapes being sought. Desimone likens it to a chorus rising above a noisy party. Individual neurons detect and fire, and then join together to force a shift in gaze toward the object sought.

▶ SEEING THE WORLD ANEW
Addressing deficiencies with vision therapy

Eye specialists sometimes perform image-based therapy to treat the complex interactions of eyes, brain, and body. So-called vision therapy has been used for a variety of conditions, including weak or missing binocular vision (resulting from poor coordination between the nerves of the two eyes); amblyopia, or "lazy eye"; strabismus, or "crossed eyes"; and other deficiencies in how patients' brains process visual sensations. Exercises may include viewing three-dimensional images to encourage the brain to process the dual eye signals that promote depth perception.

The Three-Dimensional World
Children sometimes are misdiagnosed with disorders in their prefrontal cortex when instead they have difficulty processing visual data in the occipital lobe, such as seeing in only two dimensions or failing to maintain focus. Illusions and graphics used in vision therapy challenge the brain to make sense of a three-dimensional world, by adding depth and dimension, and encourage the growth of neural pathways to process new ways of seeing.

Versions of 3-D imaging systems have existed since the 19th century, when stereographs transported viewers to the pyramids, European capitals, and distant battlefields. A wood-and-glass stereograph viewer held a card, bearing two pictures side by side, that the viewer could examine through two lenses that resembled binoculars. The two pictures were taken at the same time by a special camera with lenses a few inches apart, approximating the distance between human eyes. This parallax view created the 3-D effect. Modern versions of the stereograph include polarized images, 3-D movies and glasses, and Magic

JIGSAW GYM

Jigsaw puzzles are more than just a pleasant pastime

Jigsaw puzzles are a simple yet terrific way to give your visual skills a true workout. These visual brainteasers force us to flex our visual perception and problem solving. In addition, they are a great way to get a good dose of mental challenge.

➡ **SET UP YOUR PUZZLE**
Go ahead and get yourself a good-quality jigsaw puzzle. Look for a puzzle of at least 500 pieces (1,000 is an even greater challenge). Set up the puzzle in a space where you can leave it and work on it over time. Spend some time each day working on solving the puzzle. You can also invite family and friends to help you put the puzzle back together—the more the merrier!

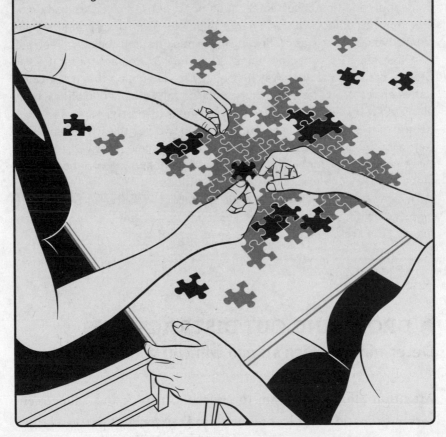

Eye stereograms—those pictures that look like random collections of colored dots until, when stared at long enough, a 3-D picture emerges.

Mirror, Mirror

Your eyes can fool your brain

D erek Steen had his left arm amputated after shredding it in a motorcycle accident. Trouble was, he continued to feel the arm—a phenomenon called "phantom limb." And the arm was in pain.

Steen's condition occurred because his brain redrafted its body map after losing contact with arm nerve impulses. It misinterpreted signals from other body parts as originating in the missing limb, making it feel real.

In the mid-1990s, neuroscientist Vilayanur S. Ramachandran tricked Steen's brain into taking away his pain by reacting as if the missing arm had been restored. Ramachandran constructed a simple mirror box, open at the top with a hole on the side for inserting Steen's right arm. The box's central mirror made it appear as if Steen had two healthy arms. Seeing his "left arm" let Steen access and fire the neurons for its movement. After three weeks of mirror box therapy, his pain went away. Mirror boxes have since been used to treat a variety of conditions.

The box underlines how the brain constructs reality out of feedback loops combining vision, other senses, body movements, and motor commands. The brain reacts to what it sees, even if what it sees is a lie.

▶ DROWNING OUT DISTRACTIONS
Determining which stimuli will win your attention

Attention allows the brain to consciously pick out salient sensory information and ignore the rest. At a cocktail party, selective attention lets you understand the conversation of someone sitting next to you by focusing on the sound of a voice and the motion of lips and face. Laboratory experiments have examined visual selective attention by having test subjects pick out words, letters, or pictures from similar images acting as background noise. The greater the similarity between the targeted image and the distractors, as between the letters O and Q, the greater difficulty the brain has in finding its prey. Research has also shown that the brain has greater difficulty as it ages in executing so-called conjunctive searches, which involve seeking two unrelated but linked visual characteristics. A simple search would target a chocolate-iced doughnut in a room full of vanilla-iced doughnuts. A conjunctive search would make the target a chocolate-iced doughnut in a room containing vanilla-iced doughnuts and chocolate-iced éclairs. That particular search requires comprehension of shape (round versus rectangular) and color (brown versus white).

Experience Trumps All

One study found that young brains outperformed old brains in the conjunctive search for a red X in a field of green Xs and red Os. However, this age-related deficit decreases if the older brain has experience with the targeted object and distractors. For example, middle-age medical technicians performed as well as younger medical technicians when evaluating x-rays, a task that requires seeking particular information amid a host of distractors. Broader applications suggest themselves. You'll improve your handling of loose change, including distinguishing one coin from another, if you practice. So too will you improve your sorting of buttons, stamps, or shoes. What you practice with your visual and prefrontal cortices, you improve.

BRAIN BOOSTER

MAP IT

Remember good old paper maps? They built our visual skills

Are you a good map reader? Those of us with visual strengths may find it an easy task. Others find map reading doesn't come easily at all, and that deciphering directions and symbols is a skill that needs practice. Also, in this GPS age, our map-reading skills can get a bit rusty.

➡ **FOR THIS EXERCISE,** take out some good old road maps. Pick a spot you'd like to navigate to, and go ahead and plot your course. Use the legend (the key to the symbols—remember what that is?) to help you figure out how long your trip will take, any places of interest along the way, and so forth. You can even try plotting a few alternate routes.

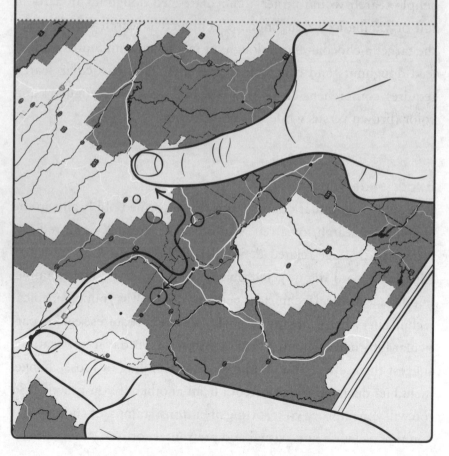

When your brain "pays attention," you choose where to pinpoint your focus. A related phenomenon called visual attention occurs below the level of consciousness. It happens as you drive, read, or interact with other people. When you're behind the wheel of a car heading down the highway, for example, your brain automatically scans the environment looking for anything requiring a reaction. It could be anything from a dog running onto the pavement to a car entering the highway via an on-ramp and inching sideways toward you.

Switching Gears

One measure of visual attention is the so-called attentional blink. It's the time required for the brain to shift from one stimulus to another one. Research on attentional blinks has focused on video games and challenges as ways to improve visual attention for young and old.

A team at the University of Rochester has found that skilled players of action video games, the kind where the player typically has to react instantly to shoot a monster or enemy soldier, have a shorter attentional blink than people who don't play video games or players who prefer slower simulation games. Some action-game players, including Shawn Green, one of the researchers, shift attention so rapidly that they lack a measurable attentional blink entirely.

Green found that action-game players can easily keep track of five objects at the same time on the video screen. Nongamers handle only three. Further investigation revealed that these differences are neither inborn nor a matter of people with various attentional blink levels self-selecting their preferred games. When nonplayers took up video gaming and practiced the high-action kind, they shortened their attentional blink.

X MARKS THE SPOT

Strengthen your ability to focus in on the things that matter

Visual scanning is a mental skill we use all the time but rarely think about. We use visual scanning to check out our world and pick out the things that matter to us in a busy scene—for example, when looking for our keys on a cluttered desk, or for our kids in a crowded playground.

Use the following exercise to challenge your scanning skills:

➡ STEP 1 Set a timer for one minute.

➡ STEP 2 Then search and see how many Xs you can find in the picture below.*

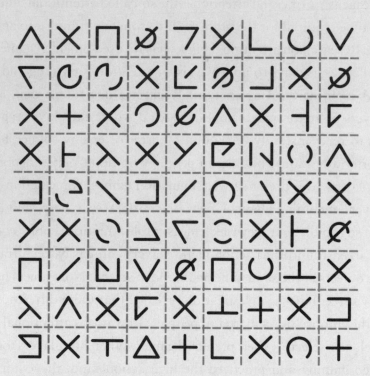

61*

Similar studies of people performing Internet searches—the manipulation of words in search engines to maximize returns—revealed that practicing search techniques increased activity in the frontal lobes, particularly in working and short-term memory, complex reasoning, and decision making.

BRAIN INSIGHT

Investigating Adderall Abuse

Some brain-altering drugs may be reaching more than their target audience

Each year, 21 million prescriptions for medication to treat attention-deficit disorder are filled for Americans ages 10 to 19. Yet some of these prescriptions are going to students without a legitimate need. Many students abuse such drugs because they help focus attention, particularly while studying for and taking tests. In 2012, the *New York Times* reported that, according to interviews with doctors and students at more than 15 prestigious schools, 15 to 40 percent of students take stimulants to help them study.

Adderall, an amphetamine that treats attention deficit/hyperactivity disorder, has become routinely abused, especially at highly competitive schools where excellent performance is a step toward admission to an elite college. A federal drug enforcement agency said Adderall abuse exists throughout the United States.

Abuse can alter mood or lead to other drugs. And, as it was designed to do, Adderall affects brain function by interfering with neurons' ability to reabsorb dopamine from the synapses. Extended Adderall use lowers dopamine levels.

"Children have prefrontal cortexes that are not fully developed, and we're changing the chemistry of the brain. That's what these drugs do," Paul L. Hokemeyer, a family therapist in Manhattan, told the *Times*.

Users apparently either don't know potential risks, or choose to gamble long-term negatives for short-term gain.

Eyes on the Road

Software and online companies have developed programs to increase visual attention as well as cognitive processing speed, memory, and executive function. Those are exactly the skills that make a good driver, so it makes sense that computer-based programs have sprung

BEAT THE CLOCK

Games that ask you to race against time build your mental muscle

Want to stay sharp no matter what your age? Try playing games against the clock.

➔ THINK FAST!
Research shows that training in these skills can us help stay more effective at them, no matter what our age. Timed activities force us to pay attention, work fast, and think nimbly—you can't beat the clock without doing so!

There are so many great brain games we can play, from board games to electronic games to computer-based, brain fitness specific training games (which have no unique scientific benefit, but can boost your stick-to-it-iveness by acting as a personal trainer for your brain). In addition, games that we play on our phones or other mobile devices meet all my criteria for getting in a bit of brain skills training.

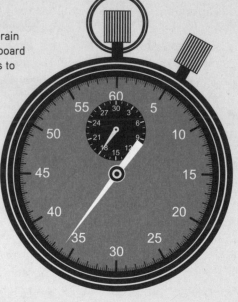

up to improve driving skills. These include DriveSharp by Posit Science of San Francisco, a visual memory system that aims to train a driver's brain to think and react faster. The manufacturer claims that people who use the system three times a week reduce their crash risk and improve their reaction time. One of the Posit Science games, US 66 Road Tour, aims to improve the useful field of view to get drivers to hit their brakes in time to avoid an accident. Players must match cars on the screen with those that appeared previously. Then, they must continue that challenge while adding a new one: pinpointing a road sign when it appears. Cars and signs eventually appear for only a moment, making more demands on visual attention.

Insurance companies have shown interest in Posit Science and other companies' brain-training software for drivers. One company, for example, invited 100,000 of its Pennsylvania customers to try Posit Science's software. Only 8,000 accepted. The *San Francisco Chronicle,* which reported on the insurance company's offer, raised a concern: Insurance companies might hold bad scores on a driver-improvement game against the players.

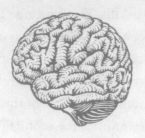

CHAPTER 7

Instant Replay

Mastering the art of remembering

When you picture yourself, you're drawing upon memory. Just as your body and brain construct themselves out of the food you eat, your concept of self emerges from your memories. Your likes and dislikes, your feelings about family, friends, politics, school, religion, and so on arise from your brain's processing of experiences. What you remember equals who you are.

Memory was once conceptualized as a mechanical process. Scientists formerly thought that memories were filed in networks of neurons like papers in a cabinet or videos in a DVD library. When you wanted to recall something, the brain opened the file or library, found the memory it sought, and played it on the viewing screen or read it on the table of your mind. Memories that faded were like lost files or locked library rooms to which the brain lost the key.

These ideas have received widespread acceptance among the public. A nationwide survey in 2011 found that two-thirds of Americans bought into the video camera metaphor of memory, and half believed that once a memory had been encoded, it would never change. Nearly 40 percent said the testimony of a single confident eyewitness should be sufficient for criminal conviction. Yet the first two statements are demonstrably false: A host of variables affects the encoding of memories, often causing distortions, and memories change over time. As for the third statement, confident witnesses are wrong about 30 percent of the time.

► A HIGH-TECH STORAGE SPACE
Memories evolve as they are stored away and recalled

Scientists now know that memory is much more complex and fluid than previously believed. For even the simplest memories, the brain scatters bits of information throughout its nooks and crannies. Sensory information is stored in the brain regions associated with processing the original sensations. Visual memories are maintained in the visual cortex at the back of the brain, while sounds (including words), smells, and other data are kept elsewhere. When you conjure the image of a teapot in your mind, you call from memory separate packets for its shape, color, size, hardness, hotness, and so on. The color and taste and smell of the tea, not to mention the tea bag, may be called up from storage, as memories tend to stick to things your brain associates with them. You might recall a pleasant tea party as a child, or that green tea is on sale at the corner store.

Once you're finished remembering something, you don't just return the memory to storage unchanged, like a library book you've kept clean and neat. Associated memories called to mind may adhere to the original memory as it returns to the neural circuits of your

BRAIN BOOSTER

MAKE THE CONNECTION

Forgetting a name or a number? Connect it to something familiar

Here's one of my favorite memory strategies: When you need to remember something new, make a mental connection between the new information and something that you already know. Meeting Florence? Connect to your great-aunt Florence, Florence Henderson, or Florence, Italy.

⬤ MAKE IT MEANINGFUL

Using the "connection technique" forces you to pay better attention to the information and makes it more meaningful to you. These critical steps will definitely boost your memory for any information you want to keep in mind, be it a phone number or a name. Try the connection technique and see how this habit can rev up your recall.

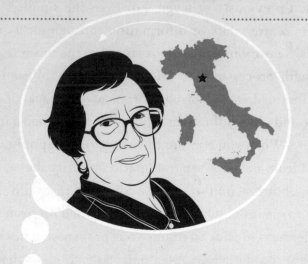

brain. In other words, the act of remembering changes memories. To use the library book metaphor, you almost always add margin notes or edit the text before you return it.

▶ THE LONG AND SHORT OF IT
Different kinds of memory serve different functions

Memory is generally categorized as short term and long term. Short-term memory, believed to reside in the prefrontal cortex, allows you to keep information in mind for a short time. It lets you know immediately where you have been, where you are, and where you're going. When you speak aloud, short-term memory keeps the first words of your sentence in your prefrontal cortex long enough for you to formulate the end of the sentence with proper grammar and syntax—delivering a witty remark, saying a solemn prayer, or reciting a limerick.

The Database Within

Long-term memory comes in two kinds: implicit and explicit, also known as nondeclarative and declarative. Implicit includes actions that are nonverbal, outside consciousness, procedural, and emotional. Explicit memories are verbal, conscious, and contextual, and are typically categorized further as semantic and episodic. Your implicit memories include the instructions your brain sends to your fingers as you type; once you've mastered the skill, you no longer think about what your fingers should do. Semantic, explicit memories include facts, the kind we think of as book learning. Episodic memories, as the name implies, provide pictures of personal events.

Knowing the 50 states is semantic memory. Remembering your visits to 47 of them is episodic.

Although remembering is a whole-brain activity, two regions play enhanced roles in remembering: the hippocampus and the amygdala, both of which are part of the limbic system. The hippocampus orchestrates the transfer of information from short-term to long-term memory. Anyone without a hippocampus, such as the patient HM mentioned in Chapter 1, forever lives in the present moment, unable to encode new memories in long-term storage. The amygdala plays a key role in encoding implicit memories, particularly those with emotional content. The most powerful, which combine encoding by the hippocampus and amygdala, are called "flashbulb" memories. They seem to capture every vivid detail, as when a flashbulb illuminates the darkness for a stop-action photograph. A personal memory encoded with great joy, sorrow, or fear gets an extra boost of encoding from the amygdala. Thus, most people remember many details of where they were and what they were doing when President Kennedy was shot, when the space shuttle *Challenger* exploded, or when they heard a close relative died.

A Resilient System

Not many decades ago, science thought of memory as a fixed process in adults. However, again and again, studies have demonstrated the brain's plasticity, or ability to rewire itself as it learns new information, at any age. We now know that older brains may take longer to process and learn new information, but once it is learned, it is just as accessible as similar information in a youthful brain.

The act of memory is plastic. It can be trained to expand and break through your previous limits.

Mark Twain's Memory Game

The famous author invented more than colorful characters

A riverboat pilot needs an excellent memory to navigate. Yet Mark Twain, a pilot in youth, notoriously forgot the "shape of a river." His absentmindedness became a joke.

Twain wanted his children to strengthen their memories. He hit upon a way to combine facts and images by driving pegs into his driveway. Each represented a British king, with the intervening spaces the lengths of their reigns. Henry II ruled 35 years, so 35 feet separated his peg from that of his heir, Richard the Lionhearted. Richard's peg was ten feet from King John's, and so on.

In 1885, Twain's idea morphed into "Mark Twain's Memory-Builder" game. Players stuck colored pins into a board as they announced a fact and date. For example, "You stick a pin in 64 (in the *third* row of holes in that compartment—'Minor Event'), and say 'Shakespeare born, 1564.' " Players memorized new dates and facts from adversaries' plays, and might eventually use them in the game.

Twain considered his game so important he put *Huckleberry Finn* on hold to develop it. But the public found the game too complicated. One critic dubbed Twain's board "a cross between an income tax form and a table of logarithms."

▶ MAGIC NUMBER SEVEN
Identifying the patterns that govern mental processing

A half century ago, Harvard psychologist George Miller found himself haunted by a particular number—"persecuted by an integer," as he famously wrote in an academic paper in 1956. That number was seven, and he titled his paper, "The Magical Number Seven, Plus or Minus Two: Some Limits on Our Capacity for Processing Information." He found that the brain can hold only about seven chunks of information in short-term memory at a time. Chances are, you can hold a seven-digit phone number in your prefrontal cortex for a few seconds after hearing it—long enough to dial accurately. But if given a ten-digit number, or an even longer one for an international call, your memory likely would fail to capture it. Unless, Miller learned, you broke it into small chunks and put each chunk in short-term memory.

Hold That Thought

When you try to hold a small group of numbers in working memory, you likely repeat them silently in your head, perhaps over and over. Scientists have dubbed this internal voice the "phonological loop." It holds sounds for a few seconds in working memory, and then drops them unless you are trying actively to memorize them. So, for example, without returning to the beginning of this sentence, you probably can recall the sentence's first three words: *So, for example*. The beginning of the sentence before that one likely escapes you— unless you peek.

Some strings of numbers make their way to extremely long-term memory through you repeatedly hearing them in the phonological loop as well as repeatedly retrieving them, which causes them to be re-encoded for storage after use. Chances are, you remember the phone number of your childhood home. And you probably committed it to memory as three chunks: a three-digit area code, a three-digit group, and a four-digit group.

MAKE A MATCH

Find that card and its counterpart in this traditional game

Maybe you played this card game for fun as a kid. As an adult, you can still build your visual focus and memory by playing good old-fashioned Memory Match:

→ HOW TO PLAY

Divide a deck of playing cards in half, taking two of each kind of card for each half.

Lay out all the cards facing downward.

Now, turning over one card in one half and one card in the other half, one pair at a time, try to find the matching pairs.

Miss the match? Turn the cards back over and try again. Keep going until you have found all the matching pairs.

Want a more modern approach? Look for computer-based versions of the game online. A version of Memory Match was recently used in a German study that found subjects who became proficient at the game boosted not only their visual memory but also their overall IQ. So go ahead and make the match!

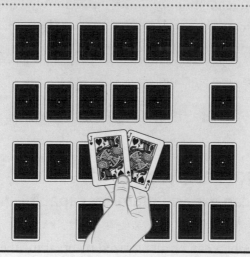

The A+ Approach

Improve your grades by learning how to learn

If you're facing an important test, you should begin preparing days, if not weeks, in advance:

Start by giving your brain the fuel it craves. Meals with plenty of fruits, grains, and vegetables enhance your ability to pay attention and think quickly. High-fat, low-fiber diets, such as those heavy with red meat, do the opposite. On the morning of the test, eat a slow-digesting, carbohydrate-rich food such as oatmeal.

▶ Study the test material without distractions. Although many college students swear they study better with music in the background, research by Professor Nicole Dudukovic at Trinity College in Connecticut demonstrates that students learn more thoroughly in silence.

▶ Test your memory again and again during review, forcing your brain to recall information upon demand. Learning things in a logical sequence—such as a chronological or geographical narrative—is more effective than rote memorization.

▶ Don't pull an all-nighter. A good night's sleep before a test helps the brain cement memories in place. Don't get up too early, either, because it might interfere with the crucial stage of sleep known as rapid eye movement, or REM.

▶ Finally, be at peace. Meditation and self-confidence can reduce anxieties, which hurt clear thinking.

▶ BREAK IT DOWN
Chunking can expand memory capacity

Very long numbers can be memorized by breaking them into chunks. But how far could an ordinary brain extend the process? How much could someone, using chunks no larger than Miller's magic number, commit to memory? In the early 1980s, researchers at Carnegie Mellon University set out to find the answer. They took an undergraduate, known in academic circles as SF to protect his privacy, and paid him to try to learn strings of numbers. SF sat and heard digits read aloud at the rate of one a second. When he started, he could only remember seven digits. But nearly two years later, after hearing those digits read aloud for 230 hours, SF could hear a string of 79 random digits and repeat it back without error. He had found a way to place the digits into long-term memory with only a modicum of mental effort. He could even recall sequences he had heard days earlier, demonstrating that his long-term memory had grown much stronger.

Give It a Personal Touch

SF received no instructions or clues from the researchers. Instead, he found his own way to make the strings of digits meaningful, and therefore more memorable, using memory cues known as "mnemonics" (pronounced ne-MON-iks). As an avid runner, he knew many recorded race times. When he heard the number 3492, he converted it into 3 minutes, 49.2 seconds, close to the world record for the mile. When the researchers gave SF numbers chosen because of the difficulty of converting them to running times, SF's performance declined. Later, SF added a new encoding method by changing some numbers to ages, such as turning 893 to 89.3, the age of a very old man.

Researchers K. Anders Ericsson, William G. Chase, and Steve Faloon concluded that the better a person could associate new number strings with things pulled from long-term memory, the more the person's memory would increase. With the right system, they said, "there is seemingly no limit to improvement in memory skills with practice."

CHUNK IT

Remember a long list by breaking it into shorter, easier-to-remember sets

Did you know that it is naturally easier for us to learn several shorter lists than one long one? This is one of the reasons that long number patterns, such as phone numbers, are broken into shorter groupings, making it easier to learn and recall them.

➲ SHORT AND SWEET

Next time you have a long list to memorize, try this simple strategy that takes advantage of our innate learning patterns: Break that long list into several shorter lists, and memorize those shorter sections. Chunking is a great technique for numbers, as well as any list that can be broken into several shorter segments, such as a grocery or packing list.

FOREST	CARPET	GUITAR
CUSHION	TOWEL	STOOL
GARAGE	PACKAGE	BOTTLE
HARE	LEMON	WHEEL

6	1	3	66	88	0	12	34	6	78
87	4	1	9	23	45	8	12	43
2	6	2	14	3	0	45	88	10
12	34	56	78	65	3	1	55	7

SF was just an ordinary guy, and not a memory expert. Journalist Joshua Foer, who also had no prior memory training, set out to learn the tools of memory experts for his 2011 book *Moonwalking With Einstein*. He began by visiting Ericsson, who had been on the team that conducted the experiments on SF. Ericsson, Foer learned, has shifted his focus to study what distinguishes experts from other people. The answer, Ericsson said, is that experts see the world in much more complex and sophisticated ways. Their expertise is not innate. It is the result of acquiring complex skills and the proper mental state to best use them. Experts improve by powerfully focusing their attention on analyzing, practicing, and critiquing their craft. To use memory experts as an example, they have broken the lock imposed on the brain by the number seven. Their method is to drink in a wealth of sensory information and relate it to vivid memories. Memory experts create rich, detailed mental images to connect to the data they wish to memorize.

▶ IMAGINE A PLACE
Using the method of loci to recall details

This may seem like a modern idea, but it is actually very old. Many people who train their memories today use a variation of a method first described more than 2,000 years ago by the Roman philosopher Marcus Tullius Cicero. Writing in the first century B.C., Cicero described the legend of Simonides of Ceos, a Greek poet who lived four centuries earlier. Simonides had gone to a banquet in Thessaly so he could regale his host with a lyric poem praising him. Something caused Simonides to step outside the banquet hall for a moment. While he was gone, the building's roof fell, crushing and mangling the bodies of the host and his guests beyond recognition. Grieving families wanted to know, who was who? Simonides found that he could identify each body by consulting his memory. He pictured the interior of the banquet hall and visualized each guest, one by one, according to the spaces they occupied. Cicero wrote that Simonides concluded that many things could be committed to memory by forming mental pictures of specific locations and storing desired facts as images placed in the image in a specific order. The order of the places "will preserve the order of the things, and the images of the things will denote the things themselves, and we shall employ the places and images respectively as a wax writing-tablet and the letters written on it," Cicero said.

The technique has the academic name "method of loci," from the word *locus*, Latin for "place." Because many who practice it use images of large buildings, the method is sometimes referred to as a "memory palace."

Stranger Than Fiction

The method of loci has two components: images representing the data you want to remember, and specific, familiar places where you store those images for recall. Here's a simple example. Imagine a building you know very well, such as your childhood home. Make a shopping list of two dozen or so items, which, for reasons unimportant except for this exercise, you wish to memorize in order. One at a time, convert each item on the list to a vivid mental picture related to the item itself. Strange and even erotic images are best because they are so weirdly memorable.

A Memorable House Tour

Put the first item at the place you associate with entering the house— at the mailbox, driveway, or front door, for example. Suppose the first item was "2 percent milk." You'd need an image that suggests the number two, the word *percent*, and milk. An image that would meet all three criteria is two bathtubs full of milk, each containing a mountain of pennies—representing the "cent" of "percent"—placed on the patio outside your front door. The image would be strange enough that it would strike you as odd, and its unusualness in a familiar place would fix it in memory.

Next, you would turn to the second item on your list into a word–picture. Let's say it's a pound of Bing cherries. You might create an image of singer Bing Crosby (or, for those under age 40-something, the home page for the search engine Bing). Have him sit on a giant pound sign—that crosshatched symbol on your phone that looks like a tic-tac-toe board—and eat a cherry pie. In your mind's eye, pass beyond the bathtubs of milk on the patio of your home, go through the front door, and place that image on the floor or furniture just to the right or left.

Next on your list is spinach. What better image could you have than the spinach-loving cartoon character, Popeye the Sailor Man, on your sofa? If you want to be sure to get fresh spinach instead of frozen, you could imagine Popeye's girlfriend, Olive Oyl, slapping his face. (He was "fresh"—get it?) Make a similarly bizarre image for each item on your list, and place them in a logical sequence throughout your house. When you want to remember the entire list, bring the first image to mind. Then tour your house in the order in which you laid out the images.

It sounds odd, but it works.

▶ ALWAYS ON
What happens when *everything* is unforgettable

Some extremely exceptional people attain nearly perfect memory without trying. Soviet neurologist A. R. Luria tested just such a subject in the 1920s. The man, known as "S" in the academic literature, walked into Luria's laboratory and asked to have his memory tested. Although S found nothing unusual in his own memory, others had declared him exceptional and referred him to the specialist.

Luria found that S remembered *everything*. After hearing the first four lines of Dante's *Divine Comedy* in Italian, a language he did not speak, S recalled every word. He repeated the lines perfectly 15 years later. Given long strings of random words, syllables, and numbers, S remembered them all, immediately and again after many years. When Luria probed into how S remembered things, he found his subject experienced synesthesia, a mixing of sensations including sounds, colors, textures, and tastes. For example, S described a voice he heard as "crumbly" and "yellow." His mind automatically supplied concrete images as he remembered things. Hearing the name of a color, for example, his mind provided a sharp image focused on that color, such as a man in a red shirt when he heard the word *red*. The complex sensations associated with each word made them memorable. When S applied himself to memorize a long list, he created his own memory palace without thinking. He created an image for each item to be memorized and placed them along the paths he walked in Moscow or at his home in Torzhok. S automatically imagined starting at Mayakovsky Square on Gorky Street in Moscow, for example, and distributed the items to be recalled at houses, gates, and storefronts.

Sensory Overload?

S's amazing memory floored Luria, but the scientist found it had its drawbacks. Photographic memory meant Luria never forgot anything, but some things are so painful or bad that they are best forgotten. Vivid memories of mistakes and painful setbacks can be paralyzing. Furthermore, S's mental images were so powerful that they competed in his mind with the reality of the moment, and he had trouble sifting important memories from those that were trivial. Past threatened to overwhelm present. S had trouble holding down any job other than one as a stage performer showing off his incredible ability. Today, he might be considered a candidate for a diagnosis of autism spectrum disorder, a class of brain phenomena linked to difficulties in social interactions and interpersonal communication as well as repetitive behaviors.

Like S, memory champions have entire subdivisions of buildings or other geographical features fixed vividly in their minds to store their memories. Each may be designated for a particular set of memories. One memory champ in Malaysia used his body parts as the topography that allowed him to memorize 56,000 words in a Chinese-English dictionary. Native Americans taught themselves long stories by associating bits of the narrative string with familiar mountains, streams, hills, and other geological features surrounding their homes.

Basic Instinct

Evolution may explain the method of loci's effectiveness. Over millions of years, evolution of the human brain has selected in favor of genes that enhance the encoding of memories of specific physical places. Remembering the places where meaty animals have been plentiful in the past, as well as how to return home after the hunt, provides a distinct advantage for survival. Those well equipped to remember topography are more likely to survive than those who

MAKE A MOVIE
Put that new piece of information into mental motion

One great way to boost our attention and remember a name or any new piece of information is to put it into action: to "see" a short movie for it in your mind's eye. Just imagine you are making a brief YouTube video for whatever you are learning.

➔ MOVING PICTURES
Keep in mind that the "make a movie" technique requires you to both visualize the information and keep it in motion. For example, let's say you met someone named Sam Waterford: You can make his name more memorable by picturing your new acquaintance fording a wide river with actor Sam Shepard or the biblical prophet Samuel.

This technique is a lively strategy for making sure that new information sticks in your mind.

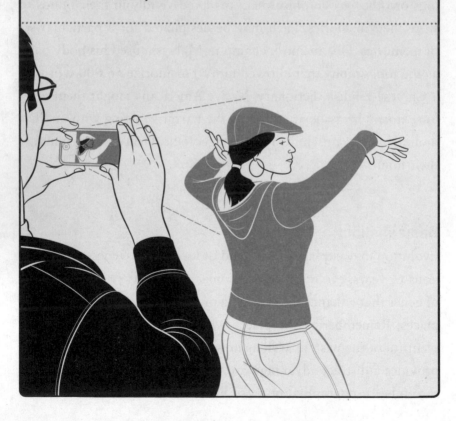

struggle with such images. The former then pass their genes along to their offspring, planting the skill in successive generations.

▶ HEY, YOU
When you can't quite recall someone's name

Evolution may also explain why some things are hard to remember. The best example is a person's name. Unless, for example, someone with red hair is named Rose, there is no logic linking a person's name to his or her appearance. Forgetting a name, although embarrassing, seldom sparks the kind of serious consequences that could prevent an individual from reproducing, and thus influence the descent of the species. Hundreds of years ago—an eyeblink on the evolutionary timescale—a name had some logic behind it. A stonecutter might be named Mason. An artisan with wood might be a Carpenter. Draper made cloth, Wainwright made wagons, and Baker made bread. Upon learning a new name and face, a learned medieval person might see the appropriateness of the name while watching a Cartwright making carts. Today, however, most names have nothing to do with a person's profession, background, or other family details. Obvious logical threads have been cut.

Memorizing names to go with faces is a part of the five-event USA Memory Championship. The other four events in 2005—when Foer observed the championship to write about it for an online magazine— were memorizing random words, a 50-line poem, random digits, and the order of a shuffled deck of cards. (The championship events were essentially the same in 2011: qualifying rounds of names and faces; speed numbers, speed cards, and poetry; and championship rounds of memorizing words, cards from a double deck, and biographical information provided aloud by five strangers at a "tea party.")

Picture This

Foer discovered that names can be made memorable using the technique he already knew of linking things to vivid images. He trained to compete in the memory championships himself and applied the method to a stack of 99 faces and names. To memorize the name Edward Bedford, linked to a photograph of a black man with a goatee and receding hairline, Foer pictured the man fording a river on a bed. The movie character Edward Scissorhands—his image called up to remember the man's first name—accompanied Bedford on the crossing.

The technique may seem strange, but it was known throughout society for many hundreds of years. Literate people learned the tricks by reading Cicero's *De Oratore* and an anonymously written Latin tract, *Rhetorica ad Herennium,* penned during the first century B.C. The nonliterate used mnemonic devices to learn long narrative poems by heart. Bards memorized thousands of verses of epic poems by relying on images, associations, and rhymes.

▶ OUTSOURCED
Exploring print's impact on human memory

Until Johannes Gutenberg invented the printing press in the mid-1400s, books were rare and, because they were hand copied, expensive. Few people were literate. Important knowledge for everyday life had to be committed to memory. But the advent of writing, followed by cheap and plentiful printed books, eroded much of the need for an excellent memory. The ancient Greek philosopher Plato lamented that the invention of writing was a thief of memory. He said writing "will produce forgetfulness in the souls of those who have learned it, through lack of practice in using their memory, as through reliance

USE CATEGORIES

Use your natural tendency to categorize as a memory aid

Take full advantage of your memory's natural learning style and use the categories technique to boost your list recall.

➡ BREAK IT DOWN

The next time you have to commit a list to memory, try breaking it into several shorter lists that belong to the same meaningful category. For example, divide your packing list by type of clothing (underclothes, shirts, and so on), or by day of travel (Monday, Tuesday, and so on).

Want another great way to use this strategy? Always depend on the same categories for lists you use again and again: Your grocery list, for instance, might always be categorized by type of food or by the aisle in the store. That way, if you forget that list at home or in the car (which happens to me from time to time!), the categories will act as a prompt for those items you need.

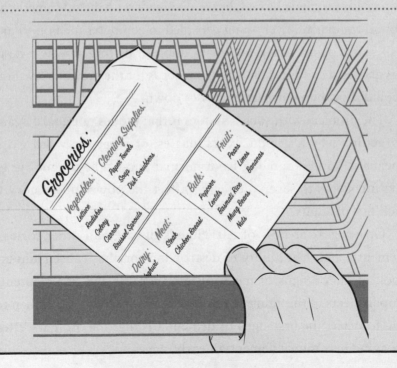

on writing they are reminded from outside by alien marks, not from inside, themselves by themselves." Learning through reading, rather than the richer experience of face-to-face discussion with a teacher, would reduce wisdom, he feared.

The Rise of Recordkeeping

Many people would argue that writing and plentiful books have freed the mind from the work of memory, allowing it to devote itself to other pursuits. A common method of bolstering memory is to fix its data outside the brain. For example, keeping all daily schedules in only one appointment book, and keeping it at hand, can eliminate many hazards of faulty memory. An extreme proponent of externalizing personal memory is Microsoft's Gordon Bell, who for more than a decade has recorded everything he sees, hears, and reads with digital cameras and sound equipment. Everything gets filed to computer memory that he can search as necessary. So, for example, if he forgets where he put his glasses, a consultation with his records for the previous few hours would show him putting the glasses down.

The problem with such a system is that it does not guard against forgetting why a person wears glasses, or what the word *glasses* means. Disorders ranging from normal "tip-of-the-tongue" grasping for words to severe dementia affect the power of memory for millions of adults.

Growing awareness of Alzheimer's disease and other forms of dementia and their ability to destroy memory has caused adults to look more for signs of memory loss than for any other potential impairments of the aging brain. One difficulty that arises when trying to detect the first signs of dementia is that the ordinary effects of aging may mimic dementia's early stages.

The Life Files

A Microsoft researcher takes the examined life to an extreme

Gordon Bell constantly updates his book of life.

Bell, principal researcher at Microsoft Research Silicon Valley Laboratory, turns every Web page he views into a PDF. He saves every email. He records and files every phone call. He makes digital copies of receipts. He carries digital video and audio equipment, including a special fisheye camera, called a SenseCam, that automatically takes a picture every few seconds.

Everything goes into computer memory. He calls his project MyLifeBits and his work "lifelogging."

Critics point out the potential privacy and security risks of making a searchable database of a person's entire life, but Bell says the positives outweigh the negatives.

"What an e-memory does, to me, is [it] gives me a really wonderful free feeling," Bell told CNN. "It's like having a multimedia transcript of your life."

The lifelog is practical. Bell tracks his diet, exercise, and physical pains to adjust his regimen, and he annotates his files to make them searchable by keyword. His brain-only memories in effect act as Web page addresses that direct him toward stored data. Bell reasons that if he forgets where he put his keys, he can find them in his sequence of digital pictures. Fortunately, he can turn his SenseCam off for minutes at a time, allowing him to use the toilet in privacy.

▶ MATURING MEMORY
What happens later in life

Some cognitive decline apparently is inevitable with age. Some is not.

A Japanese study of subjects 40 to 79 years old found that the power of memory declines more and more with advancing age. Difficulty in recalling memories held true not only for recent events, but also for events in every decade of life, exploding the myth that older memories are more shielded from decay. And that's just for subjects in a test environment who aren't under the stress of living. Elderly brains are more vulnerable than younger ones to the interference that stress, anxiety, and depression can inflict on the ability to recall memories. This can be a scary catch-22 for people wondering whether they're showing signs of dementia: As they search their memories for particular information, they may struggle because of the ordinary slowing of a mature brain. The struggle may cause anxiety, which only makes it more difficult to remember. Instead of dementia, they may just be worrying themselves into forgetfulness.

What Brain Scans Tell Us

The aging brain also has greater difficulty memorizing new information. High-tech brain scans reveal a key reason for the change. Positron-emission tomography (PET) scans measure brain cells' use of oxygen. The more oxygen a neuron uses, the greater its activation, a sign that the brain has called upon a neural circuit to perform work. When new memories are encoded, PET scans reveal heightened use of oxygen in the hippocampus.

In studies run by the National Institute on Aging, experimenters asked test subjects to observe and memorize faces. Subjects in their 60s and 70s turned out to have a lower level of activation in their hippocampus during this activity than those in their 20s. The lowered hippocampal activation correlated with the elderly subjects' greater difficulty in recognizing images of faces they had seen when mixed with ones they had not.

BE A PLANNER

Using a planner actually helps keep your brain in order

Chances are you use a calendar or planner. But did you know that your paper or digital helper may be the most critical brain tool you employ?

Planners and other memory tools get us to pay better attention and keep better track of the things we need to do. Planners help us organize and manage all the details, freeing our focus for other things.

➜ WANT TO PLAN FOR YOUR PLANNER?

Make sure your scheduler can fit all your plans in a day's entry space but is small enough that you can always have it available.

Keep in mind that no planner will work if you don't use it effectively. Get in the habit of taking five minutes every morning to check out your plans for the day. Weigh in weekly by setting aside ten minutes at the beginning of the week to review all your upcoming events and tasks.

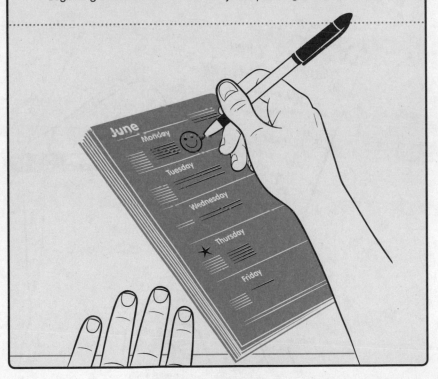

SCHOOL DAYS

Old memories may be easier to retrieve than you realize

Are you ever surprised by what you can retrieve from your long-term memory? Much of the early information we have learned, even if it was a long time ago, stays with us. Names of college classmates or our first phone number are examples of things we may remember, even if we aren't trying to hold onto them.

Although we may find our retrieval of well-learned information is slower than we might like at times (as you might experience when groping for a word in conversation, or the name of an actor), we have in general saved much in that long-term memory "bank."

➲ ELEMENTARY, DEAR WATSON

Try this simple exercise that taps your long-term recall: Make a list of your teachers from kindergarten through high school. You may not have given them much thought lately, but chances are those teachers are not as distant a memory as you think.

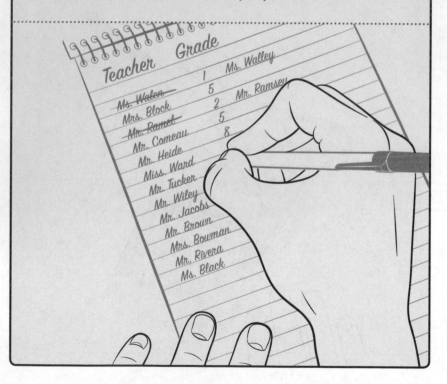

When test subjects in both groups failed to easily recall information, PET scans revealed greater activation of their frontal lobes, site of the brain's executive functions: The frontal lobes' neurons apparently burned more oxygen as the brains tried to force remembrance. However, the elderly brains had lowered levels of activation in the left frontal lobe. It was as if the elderly brains tried to compensate for the lowered hippocampal action but could not perform as well as they had in youth.

The study concluded that although memory impairment can affect people of any age, younger brains in general outperform older ones in storing new memories. Elderly brains often compensate by calling up greater energy and effort to perform mental exercises, including the recall of information. Fortunately, once an elderly brain learns a new skill, such as playing a card game or using a computer mouse, it maintains that skill as well as a younger brain.

▶ OVER THE HILL
Preparing for the onset of memory impairment

A rough dividing line seems to be age 50. Beyond that age, practically everyone has some degree of memory impairment. Scientific studies have measured this drop-off by having test subjects listen to a story told aloud. As soon as the story is over, the researcher asks the subject to respond to a list of questions about the story and its characters. Only ten minutes later—usually to the subject's amusement—the researcher asks the same list of questions and then compares the answers. The process is repeated again 2 hours later and then 48 hours after the story. Starting at age 50, the accuracy of respondents' answers shows a slow and steady decline. By way of contrast, a patient in the early stages of Alzheimer's disease loses a profound amount of information in ten minutes or less. In a similar test, early Alzheimer's subjects could only remember one or two words from a list of ten, after the lapse of ten minutes.

BRAIN INSIGHT

Alzheimer's Checklist

Learn the difference between normal signs of aging and those of Alzheimer's disease

The Alzheimer's Association lists ten signs that might indicate the onset of Alzheimer's disease, depending on severity and frequency of occurrence. If you think you have some of these symptoms, don't panic, but follow up with a medical evaluation:

▶ 1 Memory loss. It's one of the most common signs of Alzheimer's. Alzheimer's erases the memory of recently learned information or important dates or events. Increased reliance on notes, electronic devices, and family members as memory prompts also may be a sign of Alzheimer's. However, forgetting names or appointments, followed by remembering them later, can be just a typical change related to aging.

▶ 2 Challenges in planning or solving problems, such as following a familiar recipe or balancing a checkbook. Or the common task may take significantly more time. An occasional math error when totaling the month's expenses is likely unrelated to Alzheimer's.

▶ 3 Difficulty completing familiar tasks, such as forgetting the rules of a favorite card game. Less concerning is the occasional need for help operating electronic devices.

▶ 4 Confusion with time or place, particularly with things that happen outside the current moment and location. People with Alzheimer's might forget where they are. On the other hand, a typical age-related error is to forget the day of the week but remember it later.

► 5 Trouble understanding visual images and spatial relationships. Trouble reading or grasping the distance to an object or its color—all of which affect driving—may be signs of Alzheimer's. This is different from physical impairments such as cataracts, which cloud vision.

► 6 New problems with words in speaking or writing. Some people with Alzheimer's have difficulty following conversations, forget what they are saying, or struggle with the names of ordinary objects. However, trouble coming up with the right word—the tip-of-the-tongue problem—is a common result of aging.

► 7 Misplacing things and losing the ability to retrace steps. It's a warning sign when a person starts putting things in strange places, like toothpaste in the refrigerator.

► 8 Decreased or poor judgment. Giving away large sums of money on short notice might be a sign of Alzheimer's. So too might indifference to personal grooming. The occasional bad decision is a normal part of life.

► 9 Withdrawal from work or social activities. Alzheimer's may cause isolation, including spending less time on favorite sports and hobbies. This might happen when a person suffering from Alzheimer's notices obvious changes and chooses to avoid others to keep from embarrassment. A typical age-related change is the occasional feeling of weariness in fulfilling obligations.

► 10 Changes in mood and personality. People with Alzheimer's may become easily upset or fearful, or exhibit strong emotions not common beforehand. On the other hand, many people find comfort in routines as they age and become irritable when a routine is broken.

As noted, the longer people live, the more likely they are to experience a decline in memory. For most people, cognitive skills remain fairly constant, showing only a gradual decline in memory and in the speed with which they process information. A minority experiences dementia, a more dramatic, progressive deterioration affecting multiple cognitive abilities. Memory lapses no doubt cause frustration, no matter when they occur, but forgetting an appointment or a birthday is no cause to jump to conclusions about dementia. The slowing of memory retrieval is often confused with memory loss, but they're not the same thing. Usually, with time, the memories come when called. Furthermore, lapses of memory do not affect judgment or the wisdom gained from a lifetime of experiences.

▶ DECLINING MEMORY
The aging body's battle against dementia

Age-related memory loss derives from natural chemical and physical changes. One such change is the decreased flow of oxygen-rich blood to the brain that often accompanies constriction of arteries as well as the more sedentary lifestyle of the old versus the young. Others include the aging body's decreased ability to absorb brain-boosting nutrients, the body's decline in production of certain hormones and proteins that protect and repair neurons, and deterioration of the hippocampus.

Dementia's Driving Forces

Dementia's major symptoms include memory loss, moodiness, and difficulties in speaking, reading, or writing. The ability to perform routine daily tasks, a form of stored memory, also declines as the disease progresses. Causes of dementia include:

▶ **Alzheimer's disease.** It accounts for 60 percent to 80 percent of dementias and has struck more than 5 million Americans, but an absolute diagnosis can occur only when a physician examines the brain after death and notes the physical changes wrought by the disease. Alois Alzheimer, the German doctor who described the disease in 1906, made the first description of those changes when he examined the brain of a middle-aged woman whose mental faculties declined until she died, bedridden, at age 51. All brains lose some neurons as they age, but this patient with Alzheimer's had lost 25 percent of the neurons in parts of her cerebral cortex. Thick, tangled bundles of fibers appeared in many of the remaining neurons. Their presence in patients with Alzheimer's apparently interferes with normal brain functions. In addition, neurons in a brain with Alzheimer's contain clumps called plaques, which are composed of beta-amyloid proteins. Plaque buildup may prevent neurons from sharing information electrochemically, in effect isolating them from making or executing the kind of rich connections that promote complex behavior. Guidelines published in the last two years define three stages of Alzheimer's as "preclinical," "mild cognitive impairment," and "dementia." The first stage is mild impairment in which the brain exhibits physical changes but the typical Alzheimer's symptoms have yet to appear. The second includes obvious memory lapses that stop short of interfering with independent living. The third stage, dementia, brings hampered judgment and reasoning, the inability to speak clearly, and visual and spatial impairments.

▶ **Stroke.** It cuts the flow of oxygen to neurons, causing them to die. Two major types are ischemic and hemorrhagic stroke. The former blocks the flow of blood, usually when a clot obstructs a blood vessel. The latter occurs when a blood vessel in the brain bursts, often as a result of high blood pressure. This damage can impair memory and cause dementia just as surely as neurological disease. Strokes can be verified with brain scans of living subjects. They appear as dead zones amid active regions of the brain.

▶ **Frontotemporal dementia.** This is a degeneration of the neural networks in the frontal lobe. Symptoms of the disease vary widely among patients, making a diagnosis difficult.

▶ **Dementia with Lewy bodies.** Like Alzheimer's, it can only be verified postmortem. The disease causes the growth of spherical lumps of alpha-synuclein and ubiquitin protein in neurons, damaging brain tissue. Symptoms include damage to memory, concentration, and speech.

▶ **Other causes.** A host of other diseases, including AIDS, Korsakoff's syndrome, and Creutzfeldt-Jakob disease may bring on dementia.

▶ PRIORITIZE YOUR MIND
Strategies for reaching optimal health

When considering the likely decline of the brain as it ages, it is important to distinguish between two simultaneous scientific paths of investigation. The first aims to enhance or preserve existing cognitive functions. The second seeks to stave off the onset of dementia. Although the former has shown concrete results, the latter has yet to demonstrate achievements that hold up to rigorous scientific scrutiny.

Make Time for Training

A nationwide study known as the ACTIVE trial—short for Advanced Cognitive Training for Independent and Vital Elderly—raised hopes about maintaining or improving memory and other cognitive function when published a decade ago. The trial trained 2,802 participants aged 65 or older in three areas: memory, reasoning, and the speed of information processing. Participants received brain-enhancing training for two and a half hours a week for five weeks. The results indicated long-lasting improvements in all three areas covered by the training, roughly counteracting the declines that normally would be expected for most elderly people who do not have dementia.

Researchers from Johns Hopkins University and the University of Massachusetts Medical School found similar results in 2012. They performed a "meta-analysis," which analyzes previous analyses. They looked at every scientific, English-language study published before January 2010 that examined the impact of memory-training techniques. Thirty-five included a control group to contrast with the experimental group, as well as measurable gains (or losses) in memory. The study found that the most common memory-improvement method was some variation of the ancient visual imagery technique, although 71 percent of the programs relied on more than one memory-enhancing technique. Overall, the 35 studies showed an average increase in specific memory tasks. The math is complicated, but in layman's terms, the typical improvement was enough to move someone from average skills to slightly-above-average skills, from roughly the 50th percentile to the 62nd. Some memory-improvement programs seemed largely ineffective, the researchers noted.

Many experts now believe that unusual sensory stimuli, as compared with routine actions and thoughts, promote the growth of dendrites and help maintain cognitive skills. Neurobiologist

REPEAT, REPEAT

Reinforce your memory with the habit of repetition

Repetition is a simple, yet incredibly powerful, strategy anyone can use to remember better. It also is one of the most popular methods I teach, because it suits just about everyone's ability and lifestyle.

➲ MAKE IT A HABIT

The repetition technique only asks that you get into the habit of always repeating something when you are learning it. Doing so focuses your attention on the new information and gives you the opportunity to practice it. Feel free to repeat the new information as much as you need to, as this only reinforces the learning process.

Practice the "repeat" technique when learning a new name, password, or phone number and see for yourself how easy it is.

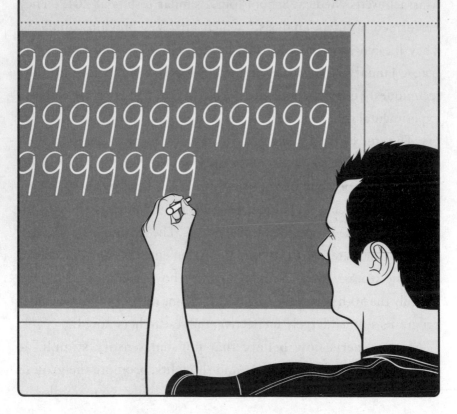

Lawrence Katz popularized the term *neurobics* for simple exercises designed to provide unusual stimulation to the brain. Examples include dialing a phone number with the fingers of your nondominant hand, carrying out a daily routine with your eyes closed, and the brain-healthy exercises provided by Dr. Green throughout this book. Memory-enhancing techniques such as simple strategies based on the ancient method of loci similarly provide unusual stimulation to the brain.

The Pursuit of Prevention

On the other hand, efforts to prevent cognitive decline have not led to clear results. A 2010 "State-of-the-Science" conference conducted by the National Institutes of Health on methods that might prevent cognitive decline and Alzheimer's disease concluded that scientifically rigorous studies have yet to conclusively demonstrate the value of *any* preventive measures. Studies of diet, physical activity, and medication "did not show any consistent benefit," said Martha L. Daviglus, a professor of preventive medicine and gerontology at Northwestern University, who chaired a panel for the conference. The strongest risk factor for developing dementia, and Alzheimer's in particular, remains age, she said. Smoking, depression, and the presence of a particular gene known as ApoE also have shown some evidence of association with a higher risk of cognitive decline and Alzheimer's.

Daviglus concluded that a regimen of mental and physical activity, including a good diet and regular exercise, combined with avoiding risk factors such as smoking, appeared to be the current best strategy to maintain brain health. That conclusion received endorsement in April 2012, in a study conducted by Rush University Medical Center.

The study found that daily physical activity may—emphasis on *may*—reduce the risk of developing Alzheimer's disease. Test subjects whose lifestyle put them in the bottom 10 percent of the population in terms of total physical activity were more than twice as likely to develop Alzheimer's as those in the top 10 percent.

Recognize Limitations, Make the Most of Benefits

What should the public make of this? Dr. Green summarizes her view this way: The history of inquiry into activities that may decrease the risk of cognitive decline, including memory loss, is young, and the science is very complicated. People should make a distinction in their understanding of such activities, realizing that some may support better intellectual performance, while others may support a lowered risk of cognitive decline, such as memory impairment. In other words, some lifestyle factors boost the good while others retard the bad, and some activities, such as exercise, seem to do both. Finally, even though the science is young, most of the lifestyle behaviors linked to good brain health, such as getting regular exercise, support good overall health. The ratio of risk to reward is all to the good.

Growing Hope

Some observers thought the 2010 State-of-the-Science report understated the case on the prospects of staving off Alzheimer's and other dementias. A year later, optimism found its way into the Alzheimer's Association International Conference on Alzheimer's disease in Paris. University of California, San Francisco, researchers presented a mathematical model that predicted as many as half of all

Alzheimer's cases could be associated with lifestyles and behaviors. That meant many people could potentially lower their risk by changing their lives. According to the model, the most important predictive variables for Alzheimer's, in descending order of importance, were low education, smoking habits, sedentary lifestyle, depression, high blood pressure in middle age, diabetes, and obesity.

BRAIN INSIGHT

Ginkgo Biloba: The Jury's Still Out

So far, claims that ginkgo extracts can fight dementia have not held up

Healers have used the fan-shaped leaves of the ginkgo biloba tree for centuries to treat blood and memory disorders. Modern medicine has discovered two antioxidant chemicals in the foliage: flavonoids and terpenoids. Like all antioxidants, they soak up cell-damaging free radicals, and thus benefit the brain.

In the mid-1990s, purveyors of alternative medicines began selling ginkgo leaf extracts as a way to combat memory loss, including disorders caused by dementia. Studies showed that ginkgo improved blood flow to the brain by dilating vessels and reducing the sticky properties of platelets. Those findings became evidence for broad claims about ginkgo fighting cognitive decline.

A study of more than 3,000 test subjects, ages 72 to 96, published in 2009 in the *Journal of the American Medical Association*, found no evidence to back up the claims. Ginkgo biloba did not slow the progress of cognitive disorders, nor did it prevent memory loss. The findings held true for test subjects who had mild cognitive problems and those who did not. A 2012 study published in *Lancet Neurology* also showed negative results.

Still, ginkgo remains popular, especially in Europe. A German manufacturer of ginkgo extracts protested the 2009 study as "methodologically so weak that it is of limited relevance," and continues to tout the leaves.

POETRY JAM

Enrich your mental library with memorized poems

Committing a poem to memory offers us a different kind of brain workout. Doing so sharpens our rote memorization skills, which we used quite a bit in school but may not practice frequently in "real life."

Such skills need to stay flexed, as we rely more than we may realize on simply learning something by heart (or head). Poetry memorization is one of the contests that make up the USA Memory Championship, so it is clearly a brain challenge worth taking on!

➲ **WANT TO GIVE OUR POETRY JAM A TRY?**
Find a poem and spend some time memorizing it. Try learning it in chunks of a few lines at a time (see "Chunk It," page 130). Need a great poetry resource? Try *www.poets.org*, the website of the Academy of American Poets. You can sign up for their "Poem a Day" program and get a poem sent to your in-box daily. (Favorite Poem Project, *www.favoritepoem.org*, features both poetry text and videos.) Or pick up a poetry anthology at your local bookstore or library. Try the poetry jam with family or friends.

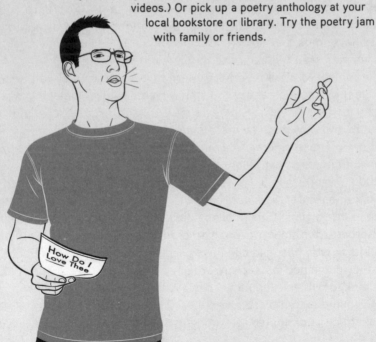

Studies at the same conference in 2012, in Vancouver, added to growing hopes. Two new early indicators of the onset of Alzheimer's were revealed to be changes in walking gait and sleep habits. And although no drug has been shown to reverse Alzheimer's, a new medication called Gammagard stabilized the disease in four patients for three years, scientists revealed at the conference. The size of the test group is too small to be significant, but much hope rests on further studies.

▶ WHERE DID I PUT THAT . . . ?
Even memory exercises have their limitations

Experts list various steps to improve memory. Some, such as doing specific mental puzzles to stimulate memory, strengthen the ability to perform particular tasks but have yet to demonstrate "generalizability," meaning improvement to all kinds of memory. Nowhere was this demonstrated more concretely, and humorously, than in Joshua Foer's book, *Moonwalking With Einstein*. Foer trained himself to become a world-class memory expert in narrow categories of competition, such as memorizing random numbers, cards, and names. Shortly after attending the world championships, Foer went to dinner with friends and then went home on the subway. As he walked through the front door, he realized he had driven his car to dinner. He had blanked not only where he had parked it, but also that he had driven it at all.

"That was the paradox," he wrote. "For all of the memory stunts I could now perform, I was still stuck with the same old shoddy memory that misplaced car keys and cars."

....

Marilu Henner's Perfect Memory

The actress is one of a few people in the world with hyperthymesia

The idea of a pill to enhance your memory has long been a beautiful dream for many with weakened memory functions, as well as an opportunity for enterprising advertisers to make a fast buck. But would you want perfect memory?

Actress Marilu Henner is one of a dozen or so people in the world diagnosed with hyperthymesia, an extraordinary memory that allows her to recall virtually everything she has ever experienced. She calls her condition a "gift."

"I don't lose my parents," Henner told CBS. "I lost my parents a long time ago and it's [memory] insurance against loss. It's the strongest defense against meaninglessness that we have."

Asked once to recall the day she got a part on the network TV sitcom *Taxi*, she said, "It was June 4 of 1978. It was a Sunday and I found out at the *Grease* premiere party."

Her earliest memory is being baptized, she said. She likened her memory searches to scanning the scene-selection feature on a DVD.

Others with the condition, such as author Jill Price, note the dark side of super-memory: Bad personal experiences linger. Unpleasant memories haunt the present. Still, Price would not give up her skill even if she could.

....

Get Moving

For everyday results, the first, and perhaps foremost, way to strengthen memory is to regularly engage in vigorous exercise and eat well. Cardiovascular exercise gets the blood pumping oxygen to the brain, and a diet rich in antioxidants, high in fiber, and low in fat provides the nutrition the brain needs. Dance appears to be a particularly good workout. Not only is it beneficial for the brain because increased respiration and heartbeat bathe the brain in oxygen, but also because learning new dance steps challenges the memory. But neuroscientists have yet to find clear, clean links between particular exercises, in particular amounts, and memory improvement.

"Right now, we can't say to somebody, 'We know that if you walk a mile every day for the next six months, your memory's going to be better,'" said Dr. Marilyn Albert, director of Johns Hopkins University Alzheimer's Disease Research Center in Baltimore.

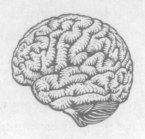

CHAPTER 8

More Than Words

Understanding mood and creativity

Your brain wants to avoid pain and cultivate pleasure. No surprise there—it shuns the sticks and courts the carrots.

But it does not grant them equal weight. Your brain has a negativity bias, placing greater emphasis on bad things than on good ones.

Blame evolution. In the distant past, our human ancestors struggled to survive. They had to avoid becoming lunch for predators while working hard to hunt and gather enough food to keep them alive—at least long enough to bear and raise children. If someone missed an opportunity for food, chances were good he or she could find some another day. But if a person missed the signs of an approaching wolf pack or saber-toothed tiger, they likely wouldn't have a second opportunity to amend the error. People whose brains were marginally sharper in their perception of potential threats survived and passed their genes for superior threat detection to their offspring.

No longer do most humans have to worry about becoming a predator's lunch. Modern threats are usually less tangible. They include war, disease, personal security (including threats to home and career), and risky social and political situations. Nevertheless, the modern brain follows its evolutionary hard wiring. People work harder to avoid a loss than to obtain a gain of equal size.

▶ THE BAD-NEWS BIAS
The brain's tendency to accentuate the negative

This difference appears concretely in the brain. Bad news depresses mood more than good news elevates it. Experiencing a single bad social interaction causes such mental anguish that it takes about five positive ones to counterbalance it and restore equilibrium. As neuropsychologist Rick Hanson writes in *Buddha's Brain,* "Your brain is like Velcro for negative experiences and Teflon for positive ones—even though most of your experiences are probably neutral or positive."

This bias toward all things negative can cause a host of problems. It generates anxiety as a kind of background noise for everyday experience. It intensifies feelings such as depression, sadness, and anger. And it can create a self-image distorted like a fun house mirror: good characteristics shrunken and twisted, bad ones inflated until they dominate.

Furthermore, evolution has vastly enlarged the prefrontal cortex of human beings compared with other animals. This region is particularly vulnerable to the negativity bias. Among other functions, the prefrontal cortex draws on remembered experiences to envision the future. It runs simulations of how a person might choose to act in a variety of brain-devised virtual realities. That made sense from an evolutionary point of view; our ancestors' brains reviewed where they found good hunting and food gathering in previous years before deciding where to go looking anew. Today, after continual growth in the prefrontal cortex, the ability to simulate choices and their outcomes has increased. Choices have expanded in modern times: Which job, clothes, food, etc., are right for you? It can become overwhelming.

Daydream Believer

The modern human brain spends a lot of time both actively and passively playing out scenarios that pull attention away from the present moment and focus it somewhere else. A Harvard University study of 2,000 volunteers in 2010 found that people spend about 46 percent of their waking hours in daydreams, not actually thinking about tasks at hand. Researchers Matthew Killingsworth and Daniel Gilbert concluded that such undirected mental video clips aren't good things. "A human mind is a wandering mind, and a wandering mind is an unhappy mind," they said. Gilbert added, "Unlike other animals, human beings spend a lot of time thinking about what is not going on around them, contemplating events that happened in the past, might happen in the future, or will never happen at all."

A lot of that mental rehearsal is channeled into visualizing negative outcomes—threats—in the future. Most of that energy is wasted. The majority of things people worry about never come to pass; meanwhile, most things envisioned as likely to bring great happiness deliver only a fraction of what the brain envisioned. But there's more impact than wasted time. Fixating on the future takes the brain out of the present moment—the here and how, where joy and love are the most real.

LIST TEN WAYS
YOUR BRAIN IS GREAT

It's easy to accentuate the positive when you really think about your brain

Take a few minutes and list ten ways in which your brain is totally awesome.

➲ THINK ABOUT IT

Why take the time to reflect on our brain's strengths? As we grow older and worry more about memory loss and other possible problems, we tend to lose sight of all the really amazing things our brains do on a daily basis. Our brains are responsible for a whole range of remarkable feats, including:

Keeping us awake (and getting us to sleep)

Maintaining our senses

Helping us speak

Letting us love

Giving us pleasure in the experience of new things, each and every day.

When we look at how much our brain does well instead of harping on small slips we all may experience from time to time, it can really change our perspective on our brain's health.

So it's important to take the time and think about what our brains do well, for a change—and I bet that you will quickly complete that list of ten items.

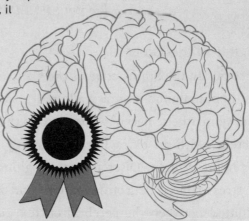

▶ UNDER PRESSURE
Staving off stress is no simple matter

Unfortunately, a great many people live in a nearly constant state of stress. Evolution once again may take much of the blame. When bad things happen, or even when you only have thoughts about bad things happening, your brain sets in motion a series of physical changes to prepare your body to deal with the consequences. If you hear a sound you recognize as signaling danger, such as the buzz of a rattlesnake's tail or the boom of a nearby lightning strike, your brain sends out a "fight-or-flight" signal to prepare your body for whatever comes your way. Something similar happens when you are rejected in response to asking someone out on a date, or when you worry about your financial future. Your brain keeps your body on edge—and that's a bad place to spend much time. In the business world, constant stress can lead to "burnout." For those exposed to stress all the time, such as combat pilots, the body adjusts and falls into a routine. But only for a while. Continual exposure tends to degrade performance.

A Jolt to the Body

Specifically, the brain activates the sympathetic nervous system and the hypothalamic-pituitary-adrenal axis of the endocrine system. The sympathetic nervous system jolts the major organ and muscle systems with an extra burst of energy and strength to prepare for fight or flight. Discrete brain regions also prompt the release of stress-related neurotransmitters and hormones. The thalamus, situated between the cerebral cortex and the brain stem, alerts the brain stem to release norepinephrine throughout the brain.

COLOR YOUR WORLD

Pull out those colored pencils and enjoy yourself

Today's the day to bring out your inner artist (even if you haven't so much as scribbled since you were eight).

➲ REFRESHER COURSE

New or different activities such as coloring, even if we do them just briefly, refresh our attention, get us to try new (or rarely used) skills, and challenge us to see the world in a different way.

What do you need to fulfill today's tip? Just go get a set of crayons, markers, or colored pencils and spend some time doodling, drawing, or sketching. You can even purchase an abstract coloring book (you can find them online) to help you color away the minutes. Go ahead and color away at whatever comes to mind.

Have kids? Share this activity and have fun together.

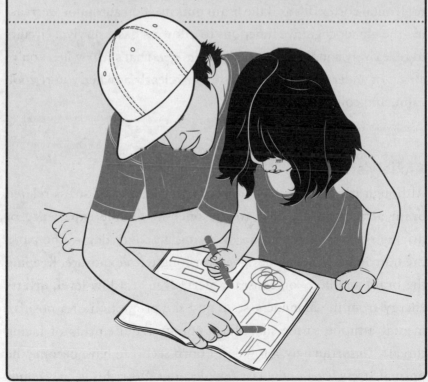

This neurotransmitter has many functions, but its primary role in response to stress is to increase oxygen uptake in the brain and sharpen mental focus. Meanwhile, the hypothalamus prompts the adrenal glands atop the kidneys to release stress hormones such as epinephrine (adrenaline) and cortisol into the bloodstream. Epinephrine increases the heart rate, speeds breathing, engorges the muscles with blood, dilates the pupils, and prompts the skin to start sweating to compensate for the increased body heat brought on by all of the other changes. Cortisol suppresses the immune system, preparing the body to minimize the impact of any physical injuries by lowering inflammation from wounds.

When all of these stress-related hormones and neurotransmitters are at work, they lower the strength of the executive function of the prefrontal cortex. It's as if the brain puts itself on autopilot, decreasing the higher cognitive functions to allow its basic survival circuits to reflexively handle any immediate danger. That's why when you're afraid or under stress, you don't think as clearly as when you're cool, calm, and collected.

Anxiety's Toll

Although it's good to have an occasional burst of stress-related brain activity in response to the once-in-a-while experience of driving on a dangerous road or facing an angry dog in the park, the human body wasn't designed for long-term exposure. Keeping the brain and body on constant alert, even at a low level, diverts energy from the immune system and the promotion of a positive mental attitude to the short-term energy requirements of facing threats. Unfortunately, a low-level burn seems to have become the normal stress level in the last few decades. Why this is so remains open for debate, but many observers point to the faster pace of life, including constant communication opportunities through email and handheld digital communication devices; increased time spent with television and video games; and less relaxation time with family and friends.

BRAIN INSIGHT

Information Overload
The age of 24-hour news may be feeding our anxieties

The decade of the 1950s sometimes is remembered as the age of anxiety. Communism threatened from overseas, from space, and, if certain U.S. politicians were to be believed, from the halls of our own government. Cold War adversaries possessed thermonuclear warheads and the means to launch them. Racial tensions exploded in showdowns over Jim Crow laws.

So why is it that Americans reported higher rates of anxiety in the 1990s than in the 1950s? Or that beginning in the 1980s, American children had higher anxiety levels than adult psychiatric patients in the 1950s?

Neurologist Richard Restak, who included those facts in his 2004 book *Poe's Heart and the Mountain Climber,* wonders whether the power of communication technology is at least partly to blame. Satellites, cable television, and the Internet constantly bathe media consumers in disturbing news from around the world. Professional communicators have capitalized on the motivating power of fear by creating advertising and marketing messages portraying a product or political candidate as an antidote. Political ads flooded TV in 2012 with scary visions of the future if the wrong candidate were elected.

"Because we are collectively feeling increasingly threatened, vulnerable, and helpless . . . our individual and communal anxiety levels are on the increase," Restak said.

HUG FIVE

Fight stress by reinforcing those emotional ties

Here's an exercise that will move your mind and your heart. All you have to do is go and give five people a hug.

➲ SOCIAL AND HEALTHY

Why this tip about getting more huggable? Studies have shown that folks who are more socially engaged have an associated reduced risk for memory impairment. In one recent study, Harvard researchers found that participants who reported lower levels of social interaction were significantly more likely to show memory problems after six years than their more social peers. Maintaining our emotional ties can also reduce our risk for emotional distress, depression, and stress, all of which have been linked to an increase in daily memory problems and dementia risk.

So go out there and get your hugs going. Hopefully this one won't prove too hard for you to do! Just keep in mind that those hugs aren't only good for your soul, they're good for your brain.

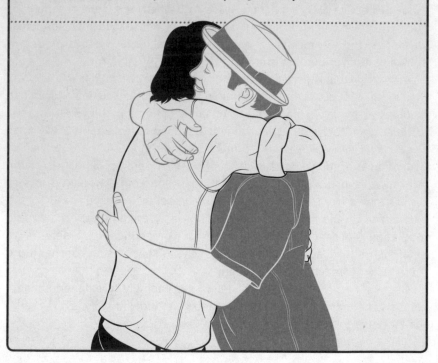

Long-term elevated stress levels can have severe physical conse-quences. These include a weakened immune system, which brings higher susceptibility to colds, flus, and infections; heart disease, including hardening of the arteries; ulcers, diarrhea, and other gastrointestinal disorders; type II diabetes; and sexual dysfunctions including decreased libido.

Long-term exposure to heightened levels of the stress hormone cortisol produces many negative effects. It encourages the produc-tion of body fat by suppressing hormones associated with appetite. It also disrupts sleep, which affects mood and cognitive function, and increases patterns of negative thinking. And it shrinks the hippocampus, the most crucial brain region for memory forma-tion. Researchers who produced a series of articles for the journal *Psychoneuroendocrinology* found memory impairment in all stages of the human life span when chronically high cortisol levels were present. Older adults with high cortisol levels during the three to six years of one study scored worse on memory tests than a control group of similar age. Among young adults, high levels of cortisol in the short term temporarily interfered with memory and other cognitive skills.

Cortisol levels were found to be higher among teenagers and younger children from lower socioeconomic classes than from higher ones. Given the relationship between cortisol and depressed thinking and memory skills, the study provides additional support for the idea that brain chemistry may be linked in part to environmental factors. And that likely contributes to the lowered cognitive performance scores recorded for children raised in poverty. Exposure to toxins and poor nutrition also may play a role. Brain regions showing the effects of chronic poverty included those associated with working memory, impulse control, and language.

▶ FIND YOUR SENSE OF ZEN
Achieving balance in your brain can help you feel at ease

A healthy brain keeps the sympathetic nervous system in balance with the parasympathetic nervous system. If the former turns the screw, the latter loosens it. The parasympathetic nervous system, sometimes called the "rest and digest" system, is the portion of the brain's circuitry that slows the heart rate and increases glandular and intestinal activity. Stimulating this system brings on relaxation and a sense of well-being.

The Om Effect

Meditation, which may affect this system, has been found to create powerful, positive changes in the brain. Tibetan monks generate electrical pulses known as gamma brain waves, cycling 30 to 40 times a second, when they meditate. According to a study at the University of California, Los Angeles, the brains of experienced meditators exhibit more folding than those in control groups. They enjoy not only greater feelings of peace and relaxation, but also some physiological benefits, including lower rates of heart attacks and strokes.

Novices get benefits too. A 2011 study led by researchers at Massachusetts General Hospital documented measurable changes in gray matter in the brains of test subjects who participated in a mindful meditation program for eight weeks. The affected regions included memory, empathy, stress, and sense of self.

Meditators have long claimed that their practice provides cognitive and psychological benefits that persist throughout the day. According to researcher Sara Lazar, the Massachusetts study "demonstrates

MEDITATE

Let go of those intrusive, anxious thoughts for a while

This activity focuses on the "soul" side of brain health. You may not think of meditation as "brain healthy," but it may be one of the best things you can do for your gray matter.

➲ **FOCUS AND LET GO**

Meditation offers many benefits. It is a perfect way to build attention, as it trains us to hold focus. It can also help us more effectively manage pain and emotional distress, all of which can detract from mental performance.

To begin, sit in a quiet spot in your house. Get comfortably seated (on the floor or on a chair).

Now, just be there, in that moment, observing your breath.

As anxious thoughts come to your mind (and they will), notice them and then just let them go. If you need help passing by those thoughts, here are two methods I have found helpful: First, just comment to yourself "everything passes," and then let the thought go. Or, as the thoughts come, think to yourself "blah, blah, blah" (which is really the noise those thoughts "make" after all), and let them go.

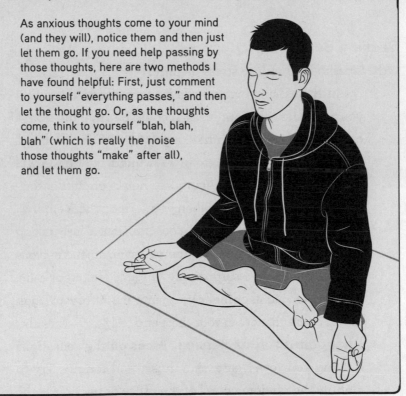

that changes in brain structure may underlie some of these reported improvements and that people are not just feeling better because they are spending time relaxing."

Any activity that focuses attention on the present brings some of the benefits of meditation. Walking, jogging, swimming, bicycling along a country road, or anything else that produces a feeling of calmness in the current moment will do. Try a low-impact exercise for five to ten minutes a day to see how your brain reacts. If your mind wanders back to stress-inducing thoughts, let those thoughts drift away so you can return your attention to the here and now. Don't keep talking or thinking about whatever it is that bothers you; fixating on the problem strengthens stress.

Seeking Serenity

Other methods to reduce stress include:

- ▶ **Visualization.** Picture a favorite place or thing that you associate with happiness. It could be anything from a cabin in the woods to a fuzzy puppy from your childhood. If you can make it concrete in your mind, your brain will activate the sensory and emotional neural circuits associated with the experience when you formed the memory.

- ▶ **Changing the way you breathe.** Consciously taking slow, deep breaths stimulates the parasympathetic nervous system, spreading a surprisingly tangible feeling of calm. Focus your thoughts on the air going into and out of your lungs, as well as the changes in your chest and belly as you breathe.

- ▶ **Sharpening your senses.** Focus on the sensations striking your eyes, ears, skin, nose, and tongue. Try to identify the random noises of the office or backyard—the laugh of a loon, the chirrup of a squirrel, the whine of a distant jet engine. Anything that fixes your attention in the present moment detracts from stress (unless the present moment is full of stressful sensations, of course).

▶ **Expressing affection.** It could be a hug or kiss with your spouse, a tummy rub for a pet Labrador retriever, or just talking about good times with friends. Social interaction improves the brain's ability to find creative solutions to problems, and physical contact appears to lower stress hormone levels as well as blood pressure.

▶ **Limiting time with video games.** Be careful about how much you play video games, and what kinds of games they are. Games stimulate the basal ganglia, crucial to the brain's experience of pleasure. It's the same part of the brain that gets excited by addictive drugs, so it's possible for a game to feel addictive. Video games that put players in stressful roles cause stress. The brain's mirror neurons fire in response to what the player sees and hears on the video screen. Therefore, if a player swings an ax to kill a monster, mirror neurons fire in the brain just as if the player had reacted to seeing a real monster, and had swung the ax in real life.

Games that simulate violence may push the brain into neural changes that don't dissipate as soon as the game is over. But the jury is out on all of the effects generated by the wide range of video games. Some games appear to reduce stress. For example, test subjects in a recent study were less likely to develop symptoms of post-traumatic stress syndrome if they played Tetris or a similarly engaging video-spatial game shortly after witnessing something traumatic.

▶ REACH OUT

Seek professional help when you're feeling overwhelmed

Decisions about treating negative mental states are best made in consultation with a doctor. Common options include prescription medications to restore neurochemical balance and therapy to adjust mental states. Both have advantages, and they are not mutually exclusive.

Medications

Prescription medicines aim to adjust neurotransmitter levels to enhance or suppress the firing of particular neural circuits. As inborn neural structure has been shown often to play a significant role in causing chemical imbalances in the brain, taking medication to restore mental balance makes sense. It's no different from taking an aspirin for a headache or wearing eyeglasses to correct vision. Nevertheless, it may be tempting for some to look upon medication as an easy fix. Use of antidepressants in the United States has increased significantly in the last two decades, making them the third most commonly prescribed class of medications. During the four inclusive years from 2005 to 2008, nearly 9 percent of Americans had at least one prescription for an antidepressant, according to the Centers for Disease Control. The vast majority of prescriptions were prescribed by doctors who were not psychiatrists for patients without a psychiatric diagnosis. That raises questions about whether that prescribed medication was always the best possible medical option.

REACH OUT AND RECONNECT

Staying social is remarkably good for your health

All of us have friends from the past we have lost touch with over the years. Here's the chance to reconnect with one of those long-lost buddies.

➔ YOUR SOCIAL WORKOUT

Why rekindle that friendship? Higher levels of social engagement are associated with better mental health. Also, being with others gives us a great "skills" workout, as you really cannot be social without staying focused, thinking fast, and keeping your mind nimble.

Staying social also exposes us to different experiences or ways of thinking, which is great for our intellectual engagement.

Finally, our brain benefits from the "intangible" side of staying social, by lowering our risk for emotional distress.

➔ WAYS TO CONNECT

In our busy day-to-day lives, it is altogether too easy to lose track of friends whose company we really enjoy. So spend some time finding that long-lost pal. Use the Internet (Facebook and Google are great tools for this), or dig out an old phone book or alumni directory. Call or write, reconnect, and make a plan to stay in touch.

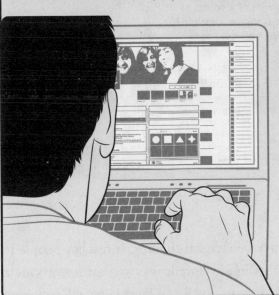

BREATHE LIKE A LION

A classic yoga exercise can help you relax in record time

Feeling stressed? Often the stress we feel can lead to a constant state of feeling overwhelmed. This kind of chronic stress can affect our daily performance, making it harder for us to stay sharp and function effectively.

➡ SAY "HA"

Here's a simple yoga breathing exercise called Lion's Breath that can help you keep stress in check in just a few minutes:

Sit comfortably, with both feet on the floor and your hands resting in your lap or on your thighs.

Start by taking a deep breath, breathing deep into your belly.

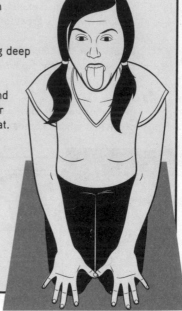

As you exhale, stick out your tongue and exhale with a bit of force, feeling the air move out against the back of your throat. You may even make a bit of a sound as you force the air out along your throat, saying "ha" (assuming you have some privacy to do so).

Repeat these steps for a few breaths.

When you are done, you will feel more alert, focused, and relaxed.

Therapy

An alternative is cognitive behavioral therapy. It teaches people to think about their thoughts in a different way so that new thought patterns rewire the brain. In her book *Train Your Mind, Change Your Brain*, author Sharon Begley describes how it works. "In the case of depression, cognitive behavior therapy teaches you to basically not catastrophize," she told National Public Radio. "So people who suffer from depression tend to take what [to] other people would be a minor setback—they had a lousy date, their roof leaks, something bad happens at work—and that gets parlayed or that avalanches into 'No one will ever love me, nothing will ever go right.' "

Cognitive behavioral therapy teaches people with depression to view such thoughts as false or as mere aberrations of the brain. The therapy patients' brain rewires itself as the patients learn to process thoughts and emotions in new ways. In the end, they have as much success bringing themselves out of their depression as those who take medication.

Begley said she has seen similar results with war veterans struggling with post-traumatic stress disorder. They may feel sharp fear or anxiety at a sudden sound, such as a door slamming, because their brains have learned to associate such sounds with danger, and those associations have formed strong neural connections over time. When the veterans received therapy in which they sensed a triggering sound or sight, but in a safe, relaxed setting, their brains conditioned themselves to quiet their fear circuits.

► BATTLING THE BLUES
The elderly are at a greater risk for depression

Depression and other negative mental states strike the elderly more powerfully than the young. Unfortunately, depression is all too common among older adults. Friends and relatives die off with the passing years, leading to feelings of loneliness. In fact, neurologist Richard Restak considers loneliness "the greatest challenge of the mature years," as half of all men and women age 90 or older report feeling lonely all the time. On the other hand, elderly people become more accustomed to dealing with feelings of loss, and many find emotional support in their circles of friends. (Surprisingly, perhaps, friends outrank family in the significance of their ability to improve an elderly person's mood. Speculation centers on the importance of confiding in friends more than family, and in the way time with friends breaks the monotony of daily life.)

BRAIN INSIGHT

Imagination Is the Best Medicine

Fictional experiences take on a kind of reality in the brain

Want to navigate through life's rapids and eddies more smoothly? Maybe your prescription should be, "Take two novels and call me in the morning."

Research in 2008 by Canadian psychologists Raymond Mar and Keith Oatley found that people who read a lot of fiction develop better social skills than those primarily reading nonfiction.

"The function of fiction is the abstraction and simulation of social experience," they said. In other words, reading about fictitious events re-creates those events in the brain. When you read about a hero's quest, your brain makes you empathize with the hero's triumphs and tragedies.

That conclusion received corroboration a year later in brain-scan research by a team led by Nicole Speer, Jeremy Reynolds, Khena Swallow, and Jeffrey Zacks. They modified an fMRI scanner to image portions of the brain activated by reading. When a test subject read about a fictitious character performing an action, the brain regions associated with executing that action became active. If the character pulled a light cord, for example, the reader's brain region associated with grasping lit up.

Neural pathways activate to rehearse reactions to potential social situations too. The implication is that if you read enough fiction, your social abilities improve along with your words a minute.

Restak believes most depression among the elderly occurs because of chemical changes in the brain. As the brain ages, it produces smaller amounts of certain neurotransmitters, and the loss alters the neurochemical balance. Compounding the problem, elderly brains also are more prone to sleep disorders, including insomnia, sleep apnea (interruptions in breathing patterns), and frequent awakening. Sleep disturbances affect the strength of memories. Restoring the brain to healthy sleep patterns and a proper balance of neurotransmitters that combats depression, often accomplished with medication, may improve mental function, including memory.

▶ THINKING OUTSIDE THE BOX
Harnessing the brain's creative power

Creativity, in the form of the desire for self-expression and inner growth, promotes physical and mental health, and appears to be particularly important for mature and elderly adults. According to Gene D. Cohen in his book *The Creative Age: Awakening Human Potential in the Second Half of Life,* creativity improves life in a variety of ways. It strengthens morale in later life, he said, by altering the way the brain experiences problems. "No matter what our actual physical condition, we *feel better* when we are able to view our circumstances with some creativity," Cohen said. Furthermore, a creative outlook fosters a sense of well-being, which boosts the immune system and contributes to overall health. It does this through the promotion of positive emotions, the ally of the parasympathetic nervous system and enemy of negative moods.

WRITE A SONG OF LOVE
Make every day Valentine's Day

It's time to expand your mind by singing a song of love.

➲ HEART AND SOUL

Chances are you haven't spent much time writing love songs. Yet, putting pen to paper and composing a tune for someone you adore is a wonderfully creative way to stretch your thinking.

Set aside some time, pull up a chair, and start composing.

Have fun as you let your imagination roam and the ideas form. Keep in mind that you don't necessarily have to perform your song. No matter how short or long, your love song is sure to be a great way to put your heart and soul into your Brain Booster.

Need some inspiration? Listen to some of the great love songs of the past. Or ask your loved ones to sing you their favorite love songs.

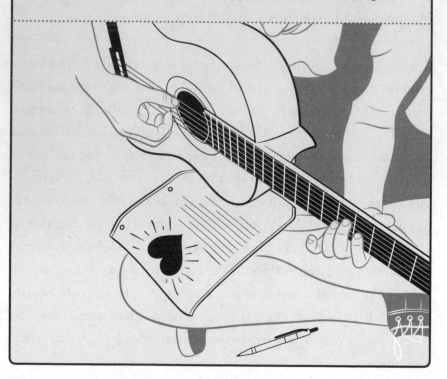

Chemical Catalysts

Specifically, biophysics and physiology professor Candace Pert of Georgetown University Medical Center in Washington, D.C., has studied the emotional impact of neuropeptides, which are released by neurons to send signals along neural circuits, but are shorter-chain molecules than neurotransmitters. Pert's study of more than six dozen neuropeptides suggests a two-way communication link between the brain and the immune system, with each influencing the

---

BRAIN INSIGHT

Never Too Late to Innovate

As bodies compensate for failing senses, brains continue to be creative all life long.

Neuroplasticity continues all life long—even in lives facing challenges in old age.

French painter Claude Monet worked to improve his craft well into his ninth decade. When cataracts began to steal his sight, he changed the way he painted—and created masterpieces of light and color at his Giverny home. Similarly, when artists James Thurber and Georgia O'Keeffe found their vision failing late in life, they developed new ways to practice their craft—Thurber by sweeping a fat crayon to create huge-scale cartoons, and O'Keeffe by switching from oil paint to charcoal and pencil.

And when German composer Ludwig van Beethoven lost all hearing at age 50, he compensated by taking the legs off his piano and setting it on the floor so he could better interpret its vibrations when he played. He also "heard" his music by clenching a stick in his teeth and touching it to his piano.

"Scientists have discovered that the brain, even an aging brain, can grow new connections and pathways when challenged and stimulated," said Nancy Merz Nordstrom, author of *Learning Later, Living Greater*. Every day that creative senior citizens used their talents to produce great works, "they were learning," Nordstrom said.

other. She believes that various body organs, including the gastro-intestinal tract, heart, and kidneys, contain receptor sites for neuropeptides. Brain-stimulated neuropeptide activity might account for "gut feelings" or "butterflies," she believes. Pert theorizes that the emotionally charged state of being in a creative zone may cause the brain and immune system to release specialized peptides throughout the body that promote good health.

BRAIN INSIGHT

Attitude Adjustment
You can consciously use positive thinking to lift the burden of bad memories

Thanks to evolution, your brain has a negativity bias. Bad experiences hit you much harder than good ones. That's your brain's way of getting you to change risky behavior. For instance, if you approached a wild animal as a child and it bit you, the experience likely remains strong enough in your memory to prevent any repeat.

Negative experiences have their place. They may promote compassion or make you angry enough about something unpleasant to demand changes. But too much negativity can harm your emotional health.

Neuropsychologist Rick Hanson argues that the brain's plasticity can reshape emotionally negative memories into more positive ones. In his book *Buddha's Brain*, Hanson suggests not only emphasizing positive experiences in everyday life, but also associating positive feelings with negative experiences when you recall them. As a memory leaves your awareness, your brain returns it to storage along with other memory strings associated with it. If you dwell on the humiliation of a particular failure, your brain stores those two things together and recalls them together. But if you can link your failure with more positive associations, such as a pathway to a rewarding new job or relationship, then you begin to shift the emotional balance of your brain.

Creativity, lack of stress, and other hallmarks of a healthy lifestyle may have contributed to the longevity of the Delany sisters of New York City, Sadie and Bessie. They lived well beyond 100 years and chronicled their century of living together in the best seller *Having Our Say.* They ate plenty of vegetables, remained physically fit all of their lives, and insisted on living as stress-free as possible, to the point of refusing to put a telephone in their home. Analyzing her longevity, Bessie Delany said, "I'd say one of the most important qualities to have is the ability to create joy in your life. I love my garden so much that I would stay out there all day long if Sadie let me. That's what I mean about creating joy in your life. We all have to do it for ourselves."

Sadie said, "Life is short, and it's up to you to make it sweet."

When Bessie died, Sadie struggled with the burden of living alone for the first time. Although Sadie once said, "I would give myself two weeks without Bessie," she outlived her sister by more than three years. In the months after Bessie's death, Sadie coped with the devastating loss by channeling her energy into the creative outlet of writing another book, *On My Own.* Sadie Delany died peacefully in her sleep at 109.

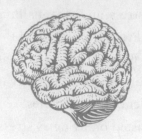

CHAPTER 9

Take Charge
Being the Boss of Your Brain

For a job that requires making important decisions under pressure, it's hard to beat air traffic controller.

Controllers must think and act quickly to keep a safe distance between planes that fly up to eight miles a minute. They must base decisions on complicated mental and physical maps in three dimensions, all the while keeping track of instrument readings and verbal and written communications. In difficult or dangerous situations, they have to parse information to focus on the most important details, and then communicate those details to pilots responsible for hundreds of lives. And although the job has its moments of boredom, controllers can never let their guard down. Studies have shown that most air traffic control errors occur during times of low or moderate activity, suggesting the dangers of failure to maintain attention.

Decades ago, when safety experts began developing air traffic control systems, they conducted an experiment simulating plane traffic. At the time, controllers gathered information from many channels at once, including visual data from video display screens, computers, and notepads, and auditory data from earphones and, if necessary, their neighbors in the room. As long as air traffic remained at a normal level in the simulation, the controllers managed the multiple information streams without incident. If one of the channels broke down, there were others to fall back on. But when the simulation stepped up the traffic and placed more demands on the controllers' attention, their ability to make decisions got worse. Eventually, the controllers lost their cool. They shouted and banged on tables, and pointed and gestured, as they tried to visually communicate with pilots who could not see them. The controllers understood the problems, but they lost the ability to make and communicate smart decisions in a timely manner. No wonder the job can be stressful. There are many variables, including weather, equipment, traffic patterns, and occasional emergencies. Controllers must decide where to pay attention; how the situation may change; and how best to plan options, make choices, and execute the best action.

► DECISIONS, DECISIONS
How the brain performs higher level thinking

Although the technology of air traffic control has improved and now places fewer demands on controllers' attention, it's still a job, like many, where decision making remains crucial. Angelika Dimoka, director of the Center for Neural Decision Making at Temple University, has scanned the brains of test subjects urged to make difficult decisions based on multiple variables. She chose an airport-related scenario, the purchase of landing slots. Her test subjects bid on slots that could be bought singly or in bundles, in a wide array of combinations. Bidders had to juggle not only prices—they aimed to get the best deals at the lowest cost—but also such variables as weather, the schedule of connecting flights, and passenger load. As the test subjects had to simultaneously weigh more and more information while making decisions, fMRI scans showed heightened activity in their dorsolateral prefrontal cortex. This brain region behind the forehead not only plays a key role in making decisions, but also helps regulate emotions and orchestrates other higher-cognitive functions.

At some point, the addition of extra information acted like the straw that broke the camel's back, causing activity in the dorsolateral prefrontal cortex to drop dramatically. The test subjects couldn't make smart decisions, and they struggled to control their frustration. "With too much information, people's decisions make less and less sense," Dimoka said.

▶ UNPLUGGING
Strategies for coping with today's surplus of stimuli

Dimoka's findings are bad news for the millions of people continually and intimately connected with information streams, such as the words, numbers, pictures, videos, and more available on the Internet and digital handheld devices. Information overload is a reality that is only likely to get worse.

One way to fight back is to relax the mind.

The brain increases its ability to solve difficult puzzles when it shifts its attention away from a problem and turns inward. This can create a catch-22: If you've ever obsessed about finding the answer to a thorny issue at work or in your academic studies, you

BRAIN GAME NIGHT

Join with friends to take on some brain challenges

Have you got game? You certainly should, it's good for your brain! Try a Brain Game Night to get your game going.

➲ GOOD COMPANY

We know that mental activity is a key ingredient in any brain fitness plan. In addition, staying social has been found to reduce your risk for memory loss over time. What better way to get a good dose of both than having a brain game night with family or friends?

You can play board games, do jigsaw puzzles, or play some old-fashioned charades or Pictionary. This is a time to put away electronics and engage in some real-world interactions. Brain Game Night can be a wonderful time to pass down the rules of some favorite, tried-and-true games, as well as to try some new ones. Or try holding your own college bowl (remember those?) and test your knowledge of facts in all sorts of categories. Enjoy the company while giving your brain a workout!

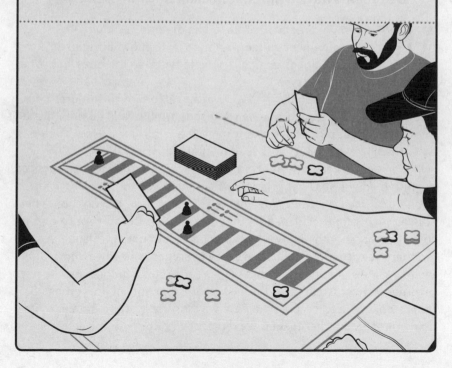

probably find it difficult to *force* your mind to relax by *ordering* it to do so. But relaxation often comes quietly on its own when the brain is cut off from an overload of sensations. A pleasant shower or comfortable period of meditation may subtly push the brain into a state that stops the aggravating sensations brought on by too much attentional focus. Psychologist Joydeep Bhattacharya at the University of London says, "That's why so many insights happen during warm showers."

BRAIN INSIGHT

Sweet Dreams

Do dreams have a purpose? Scientists still aren't sure

Why do we dream? Everyone has dreams, although not everyone remembers them. And it's extremely difficult to keep people from dreaming. Those facts raise the question: What function do dreams serve?

Sigmund Freud, founder of psychoanalysis, believed the brain conjured dreams as a way to access repressed wishes and desires. It's an interesting idea, but a hard one to test in a laboratory: How does one scientifically examine a repressed mental state?

Modern observers are split on the role of dreams. Some, such as cognitive scientist Owen Flanagan, author of *Sleep, Dreams and the Evolution of the Conscious Mind,* believe dreams have no function whatsoever. According to Flanagan, they are a side effect of sleep and its role of recharging the body—"nothing, nada, just noise," Flanagan said.

Others see dreams as the brain's way to process the day's information, including the sorting of data into memory's circuits. In this view, the act of dreaming contributes to the necessary function of forgetting. Still others believe dreams create a safe way for the brain to simulate life's many threats as a therapeutic way to deal with them.

You Are Getting Sleepy . . .

Bhattacharya discovered a link between the phenomenon of insight and a steady brain rhythm emanating in the right hemisphere, as registered on an electroencephalograph, or EEG. The EEG records brain activity in the form of electrical impulses. These impulses move through the brain in a variety of frequency ranges, like radio stations arrayed throughout the AM and FM radio bands. The lowest frequency, seen in delta waves, is most commonly found in brains in a state of deep sleep. In ascending order above the delta waves are theta waves, which occur during prayer, daydreaming, and some sleep stages; alpha waves, associated with feelings of calm and control; beta waves, common in active mental states such as analyzing problems and making decisions; and gamma waves, which occur all the time in nearly all brain states and may play a role in synthesizing various brain functions. What Bhattacharya found is that the onset of alpha waves in the right-hand lobes heralds the *aha!* moment when the brain solves a nagging problem. His tests have shown that people who cannot reach a threshold level of alpha waves cannot solve tricky word problems even when given heavy hints.

Small wonder, then, that in a German study involving word puzzles that required a flash of insight to solve, subjects who reported feeling happy—the positive, calm mood typical of alpha waves—outperformed those who reported negative moods. Cognitive neuroscientist Mark Beeman at Northwestern University even found that people performed better at solving insight puzzles after watching a video clip of comedian Robin Williams, which apparently lightened their mood and helped them relax. Beeman has linked insights to the relaxed period typically experienced in the first few moments after waking up. In its drowsy, discombobulated state, the morning brain is ideally suited for solving mental puzzles by not actively focusing on them.

PRACTICE MINDFULNESS
Learn to live in the moment

As we rush through our day, we often miss important details and meaningful moments. All this busy-ness takes a toll on our brain health. Wouldn't it be nice if we could just slow down, learn to be more focused, and give more attention to what we are doing?

➜ ACTIVE MEDITATION
The practice of mindfulness asks us to do just that. Becoming more mindful simply requires us to be more in the moment of our experience. Doing so regularly helps us build focus and concentration, provides stress relief, and helps us capture more important moments that we might otherwise miss. In fact, mindfulness is an active meditation practice that carries the same benefits as meditation for our everyday intellectual functioning and long-term brain health.

➜ PICK A TARGET
Begin to practice mindfulness by targeting certain times or actions. Become more aware through all your senses of something in your daily life, such as the first bite of each meal or your daily walk to work. Becoming more mindful will help both your mind and your spirit.

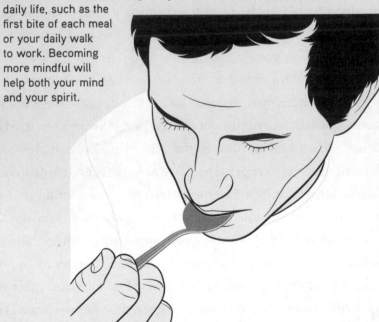

This suggests a practical way to try to trick your brain into doing its best work. If your mornings typically are overloaded with tasks to get done before work or school, try setting your alarm clock to give yourself just a few minutes of quiet time before you have to begin your responsibilities. When the alarm bell rings, hit the snooze bar but don't go back to sleep. Try thinking in a half-awake state.

► THE EXECUTIVE IN YOUR HEAD
Taking command of your body and your life

Making good decisions and taking control of your mind are important skills. Fortunately, your brain's cognitive control center, the prefrontal cortex, is not hardwired. You have a strong measure of control over what you think, and what you think about it. In short, you can be the boss of your own brain.

Be Selective

Your ability to make choices is good for your health. People who are cared for by others often show concrete improvement if they are given the opportunity to make decisions affecting their lives. Even relatively insignificant decisions, such as which shirt to wear or when to eat, boost the health of residents in nursing homes and other care facilities. And people thrust into traumatic situations, such as a bad accident or a natural disaster, usually have less significant suffering in the long run if they made decisions at the time of the trauma and acted on them, such as the choice to comfort victims.

FIVE USES FOR MASKING TAPE

Think outside the box by finding new uses for familiar items

One measure of intellectual nimbleness is our ability to solve problems by thinking creatively, nimbly, and out of the box. So here's a little problem for you: What can you do with masking tape?

➲ STRIVE FOR FIVE

Think of at least five uses for the tape. Clearly, masking tape can attach one object to another—can you think of five other ways to employ it? Or even a few more?

If you like this exercise, try thinking of the many ways you can use the following household items:

Paper clip

Lemons

Paintbrush

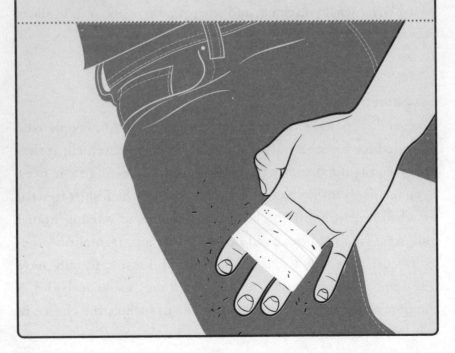

You can exercise control not only over how to act, but also about how to think and feel. If you choose to have positive feelings and attitudes, you'll be doing your health a favor.

Scientists at the Wageningen University in the Netherlands interviewed nearly 2,000 elderly men and women and classified them as optimists or pessimists by whether they agreed with statements such as "I still have many goals to strive for." The researchers followed up with their interviewees nine years later. Those who had expressed optimism in the initial interviews had far lower death rates than their more pessimistic peers—63 percent lower among the men, and 35 percent lower among the women.

The Dutch study controlled for other factors that could have influenced the subjects' longevity. These included whether the interviewees smoked or drank alcohol, as well as their weight, diet, and amount of physical activity. Researchers found a strong correlation between optimism and health-promoting behavior, such as eating and exercising well. It was as if the test subjects who felt good about their futures worked to ensure they would be there to enjoy them. Perhaps optimism increases the will to live. Another theory suggests that greater social interaction of optimists, as opposed to pessimists who wish to be left alone, promotes longevity by lowering levels of the stress hormone cortisol. The payoff at the end of life, according to University of California researchers: Optimists live about seven and a half years longer than pessimists.

The Rewards of a Glass-Half-Full Mentality

But optimists don't have to wait until old age to enjoy benefits. Being optimistic brings immediate returns. According to researchers at Carnegie Mellon University in Pittsburgh, optimism strengthens the ability of the body's immune system to fight off disease and also offers protection against the negative effects of stress. Other studies have shown that optimists suffer less chronic pain and have fewer disabilities than pessimists.

Take It up a Notch

Constant challenge will keep you on top of your game

If you want to improve a skill such as playing guitar, choose to get out of your comfort zone.

Most practiced physical actions, such as hitting a golf ball or shooting a free throw, occur as the brain is in or near a state resembling autopilot. The first time you shot a free throw, fingered the notes in a G chord, or swung a seven iron, you probably used your frontal lobes to concentrate on the required motions. As you made mistakes, you kept your level of concentration and made adjustments. But at some point, you likely became satisfied, and your improvement stopped. The neural processes associated with the skill then migrated from the front of the brain to the back, to the cerebellum.

To achieve your potential, move the skill back up front, to the frontal lobes. Try challenging yourself. If you're a musician, practice the toughest part of a song until you've mastered it. If you play sports, try to swish those free throws or drop your tee shot into a small circle. Analyze the motions that make up the skill and adjust. And don't just do it one day. True experts practice both deliberately and continually.

A general sense of well-being also improves cognitive function. Attitudes sometimes can become self-fulfilling prophecies. For example, if you believe you will do well on a test, you will perform better than if you believe you will do poorly. This was demonstrated by a North Carolina State University study of adults ages 60 to 82. The researchers gave the same mathematical and memory tests to the entire group, but before beginning, they dropped hints among members of one subset that their age might negatively affect their performance: They said the test measured how age affected memory, and asked them to write their age just before taking the test. Group members reminded of their age and the likelihood of it affecting test results performed worse than those who simply took the test. The difference was more pronounced for the youngest members of the group, as well as those who had the highest education levels. The researchers speculated that the oldest test subjects showed less impact from the experimental treatment because they felt secure in who they were and cared less how others defined them.

These findings prove true the words of the Stoic Greek philosopher Epictetus, who lived nearly 2,000 years ago: "Men are disturbed not by things but by the views which they take of them," he said. But if you're not an optimist and want to become one, what can you do? Changing a core component of one's personality isn't as easy as flipping a switch. Neural pathways fire more easily after they have been fired often because synaptic connections grow strong for routines. So, if you have lived for years reacting with anxiety, stress, doubt, and cynicism to whatever comes your way, your neural pathways have figuratively become four-lane interstate highways for negative mental states.

▶ POSITIVE VERSUS NEGATIVE
Using the cognitive principles to change your attitude

The tools of cognitive therapy can help switch attitudes from negative to positive by injecting the concept of choice, or decision making, into mental states. Cognitive therapy rests on a foundation of three principles. First is to agree with Epictetus: The way you choose to view events in your life is crucial to your mental states. Second is the close relationship between moods and thoughts: Altering one alters the other. And third is that by manipulating thoughts, which can be managed to a degree, you can manipulate your moods.

The Choice Is Yours

The first principle suggests that you have a choice in how to view what happens to you. Although it may not seem true at times, it always is. Thus, when something bad happens to you, you can choose to try to recast it by looking at it in a new way that emphasizes potential good. If you're underperforming at work, it might be because you devote so much time to family, children, church, or something you rank even more important. If you lose your job, it might be the opportunity to seek a new career that you have wondered about, but never had the courage (or time) to explore. If you cannot afford an expensive vacation far away, you might learn to better appreciate the attractions in your own county or state. And if your car needs to be in the repair shop for a couple of weeks, you might discover that you like to bike, walk, or carpool. This is not the same as being a Pollyanna. Sometimes there is no bright side. But there are always other perspectives, and it's beneficial to seek them out.

The Snowball Effect

The second principle probably calls to mind examples from your own life. If you've been in a bad mood, you likely recalled memories of bad things that happened in your life. Or, if you get a piece of bad news, such as a phone call telling you of a loved one who has been hospitalized, your mood probably went dark in a hurry. That bad mood may have triggered more negative thoughts, because moods and thoughts reinforce each other, like a feedback loop in an amplifier. For example, if you think you performed poorly on a college exam, you might feel depressed or angry. That might trigger thoughts that you don't belong in a particular college class, or that you're not as smart as your classmates. That could eventually lead to thoughts such as, "I'm no good at anything." That blanket statement is a long way from getting a less-than-desired grade on a single test, but that's a common neural pathway that some brains have established over time.

Look for the Silver Lining

The third principle is the key to healthy mental states. Recasting how you think about something sets off a new chain of thought–mood–thought reinforcement. If you get a bad grade, for example, don't think, "I'm stupid." Instead, embrace the perspective, "Everyone makes mistakes. Everyone bombs a test once in a while."

Negative thoughts to be avoided arise in common categories. These include:

▶ Black-and-white thinking. Few things are wholly good or bad, but it can be easy to see them that way. And no relationship is without occasional problems.

▶ Exaggerating and overgeneralizing, which are similar to black-and-white thinking. Don't say, "I never have any fun," or "You never listen to me."

▶ Predicting worst-case scenarios that aren't likely to come true. Don't misinterpret a sneeze as anything more than a sneeze, unless you really are sick. Don't believe one mistake will forever change your relationships.

▶ Rationalizing good things that happen as if they weren't truly good. Don't try to read other people's minds when they interact with you, looking for selfish motives for good deeds. Accept good deeds with good cheer.

▶ Personalizing problems that aren't the fault of any one individual. Nobody is the center of the universe.

Rules of Perspective

Cognitive therapist Gillian Butler and psychiatrist Tony Hope, authors of *Managing Your Mind: The Mental Fitness Guide,* offer four "rules of perspective" to help you skirt destructive thoughts that set off the feedback loop of negativity. First is the so-called "100-year rule." When something bad happens, ask yourself whether it will matter in a century. The exercise forces the new perspective of seeing events from a great distance—which almost always makes them look small.

Second is the "measuring rod rule," which invites you to ask yourself whether something bad in your life truly is the most important thing in your life. So what if you wrecked your car—you can get another one, and you have other things that are more important.

Third is the "middle of the night" rule. It suggests that dark moods and thoughts flourish in the nighttime, but the clarity of daylight often brings another view.

And the final rule is the "statute of limitations." Don't worry about things long after they could possibly continue to have substantial impact. Stop punishing yourself. One way to let go of old problems is to reimagine them as if they belonged to somebody else.

HONORABLE OPPOSITION

Shake up your mental routine by taking a fresh point of view

This tip asks you to open your mind. Often we fall into the rut of listening only to information and opinions that affirm the beliefs we already hold, be they in our political, philosophical, or personal lives. Listening to the opposite point of view can help us to rethink our positions (though not necessarily change them!), giving us a chance to engage our minds in a way we may not have done in quite a while and perhaps even see things from another's point of view.

➲ LEAVE THE COMFORT ZONE

Spend some time today tuning in to TV or radio stations or reading articles that hold the opposite point of view from your own. Try talking about what you read with friends or family, seeing if you can even hold the counter position in your discussions.

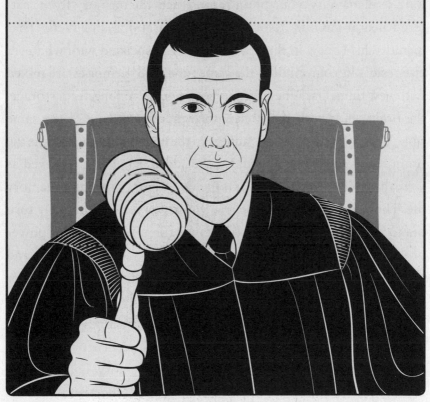

▶ REVISITING THE PAST
How memories can alter your mood

This ability to choose affects not only the brain's view of what's happening now, but also how the brain handles memories. Even old memories can be recast in a more positive light.

When a memory forms, your brain stores some significant details and trashes the rest. Along with those details, emotional colors are stored as well. Thus, your memories of a childhood picnic may include not only where your family gathered and what they ate, but also how you felt at the time.

Memories are fluid, not fixed. When you recall something from long-term memory, your brain reconstructs the memory from scattered neural circuits associated with sensations and facts. That memory, held anew in the brain, then gets associated with whatever else resides in your mind at the same time. Old memories are mixed with new thoughts. When the memory returns to long-term storage, the brain sends with it any new thoughts that it held at the same time. These new associations adhere to the memory. The next time the brain recalls the original memory, the added details are retrieved as well; the brain treats them all as if they were part of the same memory file. Thus, many things you believe you know for certain likely turn out to be at least partly false upon examination. That's why the power of suggestion can change memories or even create false ones, and why some eyewitnesses crumble under cross-examination in court or provide credible testimony that later proves to be mistaken.

If you create negative mental states such as sadness or anxiety whenever you call up a memory from long-term storage, those dark feelings slowly become glued into the memory. For example, if recalling a date in high school leaves you sad, the neural circuits encoding that sadness grow stronger. Do it often enough, and you will physically change the power of the synaptic connections in your neural circuits.

WHAT'S IN THE CLOUDS?

A childhood pastime is still enjoyable and good for your brain, too

Remember this game from childhood? It's still fun, and even offers your brain a bit of recharge by helping you to flex your abstract reasoning skills.

⮕ LOOKING UP

Go outside on a partly cloudy (or partly sunny) day. Pick a nice spot where you have a good view of the sky and passing clouds. Next, take some time to see how many different things you can find in the clouds. You can look for shapes, objects, faces, animals, or even clouds that remind you of someone you know. Challenge yourself to find new things in the same formation as the clouds shift over time.

Want to make it more fun? Go ahead and do it with someone else.

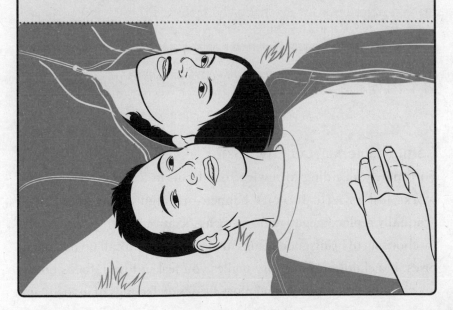

The Age of Reason

Your brain is not physically mature until you are in your 20s

Turning 18 is more or less the magic moment when people are expected to take full responsibility for their actions. In America, this includes receiving the right to vote, use tobacco products, and, generally, be emancipated from parents and handle finances.

But 18 isn't the age of perfect reason.

The brain's maturation includes the gradual spread of a pale, waxlike substance called myelin around axon fibers. Myelin acts like electrical insulation, increasing the speed and efficiency of information-sharing among neurons. If your brain were a digital connection, myelin would boost your bandwidth.

Myelination begins shortly before birth and isn't complete until early adulthood. It begins in the motor and sensory regions toward the back of the brain and works its way forward. Last to become fully myelinated, sometime in the third decade, is the prefrontal cortex, center of reason and control of behavior. Men complete myelination later than women.

Nowhere is the immaturity of a young adult's brain seen more clearly than in automotive statistics. In England, men aged 17 to 20 account for one third of all convictions for dangerous driving, despite being only 3 percent of drivers. Small wonder insuring a driver under age 25 is so expensive.

Comfortable in Your Own Skin

Fortunately, deciding to rewire your brain in a more positive way works just as well. It won't happen overnight. Instead, you can gradually replace negative memory associations with positive ones by choosing to bring good things to mind when you call up bad memories. If a childhood memory makes you feel unloved, focus on the love around you today. If a memory brings on feelings of inadequacy, think about something you're proud to have accomplished, and let it sink in. Then, over the next hour or so, try to repeat the connection between positive associations and the original memory. Research by behavioral neuroscientist Marie Monfils at the University of Texas suggests that in the moments after recalling a memory, the brain has greater power to change negative ones than positive ones.

In addition to thinking good thoughts, it helps to overtly state positive things to yourself out loud or in your mind. You don't have to be the goofy, saccharine character Stuart Smalley from *Saturday Night Live* ("I'm good enough. I'm smart enough. And doggone it, people like me."), but it wouldn't hurt to emulate Fred Rogers, the soft-spoken educator and Presbyterian minister beloved by two generations of children for his years on the Public Broadcasting Service program *Mister Rogers' Neighborhood*. He nurtured self-worth, telling children, "You always make it special for me by just your being you. I like you just the way you are. You know that, don't you?" And then he told children he would see them the next day, a promise that no matter what, his relationship with them would continue.

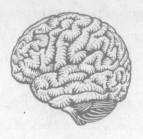

CHAPTER 10

···

Live Smart
Nurturing your whole body

Much of the advice of this book has focused on specific tasks or challenges you can use to improve the health of your brain or those of your loved ones. These range from learning to speak a second language or play a musical instrument, to training your memory with the method of loci, to doing word and number puzzles. Although these exercises all have value, research suggests they may not be as important as the simple, everyday care and feeding of body and brain through proper diet, exercise, sleep, and protective measures against brain injury. These may seem like small steps. But they add up. Nothing is better for your long-term brain health than having a strong body shaped by eating the right foods, following a regular exercise routine, and otherwise ensuring that your brain gets what it needs and avoids what it doesn't. Specific nutrients are absolutely key to keeping the brain in good shape, but too much of a good thing is bad. A balanced diet should include a wide variety of foods yet limit sugar, caffeine, alcohol, and other substances beneficial in small amounts but harmful in large ones.

▶ FEED THE MACHINE
Providing your brain with adequate nutrients

The brain is a furnace burning energy, consuming about a quarter of all the body's blood sugar and oxygen. Yet the brain has no way to store extra fuel when supplies run low. Without proper nutrition and ample water, the brain grows sluggish and eventually begins to shut down.

The Bittersweet Truth About Glucose

The brain's main fuel is glucose, also known as blood sugar. Not enough glucose in the bloodstream impairs mental focus, the ability to learn new information, and the ability to retain it. So, your mother was right—you should eat a good breakfast before heading to school in order to raise your glucose level. But if your breakfast, day after day, contains abundant sugar on your cereal or in your coffee, your body will compensate for the overdose by pumping out more insulin. Too much in the bloodstream subjects the brain to oxidative stress and inflammation, aging the brain prematurely. Meanwhile, elevated glucose levels not only add to the likelihood of increased body fat, but may also shrink the hippocampus, which regulates the functions of memory. According to recent research at Columbia University Medical Center, even moderately high levels of blood sugar can reduce blood flow to the hippocampus and contribute to cognitive deficiencies.

ALCOHOL CHECK

Drinking can make it harder for you to learn and remember new facts

At a family reunion or business event, and want to make sure you remember new names and faces? Try limiting how much alcohol you drink.

➔ THINK BEFORE YOU DRINK
Alcohol is known to impair the ability to learn new information. In addition, as you grow older, you become more vulnerable to the effects of substances like alcohol, because your body doesn't process such substances as quickly as when you were younger.

Keep an eye on how well you balance your alcohol intake, especially at times when remembering new information, such as names, is critical. Increase your awareness of how drinking may be making it harder for you to remember, and control your consumption.

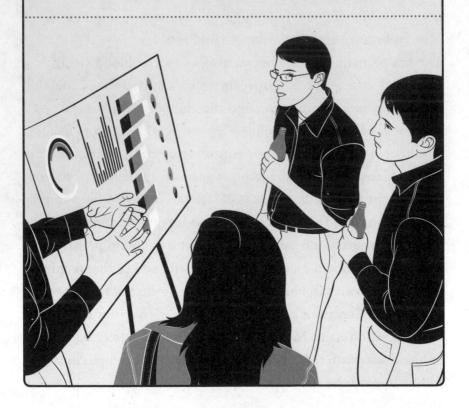

The calorie-rich lifestyle in the United States adds not only to the growing incidence of obesity but probably also to the increase in mental disorders in old age, when the brain loses some of its ability to regulate glucose levels. That's bad news for those with a Santa Claus-like physique. Belly fat doesn't just benignly jiggle; it actively releases streams of damaging inflammatory cells and hormones into the bloodstream. A 2008 study by Kaiser Permanente in California indicated that these fat-brewed chemicals play a role in the onset of some dementias. The Kaiser Permanente researchers dug into the medical records of people who were in their 40s in the 1960s and 1970s, and then tracked their health three decades later. In their 70s, at the time of the follow-up, people in the original group who had large waistlines and were obese, an indicator of the presence of abdominal fat, were more than three times as likely to have been diagnosed with dementia than those who had maintained a slim physique.

▶ YOU ARE WHAT YOU EAT
How nutrition affects outlook

You should not only consume the proper amount of calories, but also get the right kind. Nutrients provide the molecular building blocks to create and replenish the brain's stocks of neurotransmitters, the chemicals that carry electrical signals between neurons. Deficiencies can cause mood changes, confusion, memory loss, and other mental disturbances. At times, mental problems that appear to be associated with dementia or other diseases are merely temporary manifestations of poor diet or lack of proper blood circulation.

Consider mood. The neurotransmitter serotonin prompts feelings of serenity and fights depression, anxiety, and inability to sleep.

Eating carbohydrates such as pasta causes an amino acid called tryptophan, which the body needs to make serotonin, to enter the bloodstream via the gastrointestinal tract. Failing to get enough tryptophan into the bloodstream can lower mood significantly, and can contribute to chronic depression if the condition persists. Equally crucial to keeping mood elevated are vitamins and minerals. Psychiatric patients often have lowered levels of vitamin C and B-complex vitamins, including folic acid, which the body uses to make oxygen-carrying red blood cells.

A Diet Every Part of You Can Appreciate

Diets that support overall health and are good for your heart will also be good for your brain. They would include the following practices:

▶ **Eating a variety of foods to cover the spectrum of nutrients.** There is no one "perfect" food. Perfection comes from eating many kinds of foods. Consider a "Mediterranean diet"—with a focus on plant-based foods, fish and poultry, olive or canola oils instead of butter, and herbs and spices instead of salt. Try to cover half of your plate at every meal with vegetables of different colors to get not only fiber but also vitamins and minerals. Also eat fruits and nuts, the latter of which provide a good source of protein. Meat has plenty of protein, but like sugar, it should be eaten in small amounts—or avoided entirely, if you can manage to become a vegetarian. A diet rich in meat, particularly fatty red meat, has been linked in multiple studies to higher incidence of heart disease and cancer.

▶ **Eating foods rich in antioxidants.** These chemicals soak up bandit molecules called free radicals. Natural by-products of oxidation, the body's metabolism of oxygen, free radicals have at least one unpaired electron in the shells of their atoms. This creates an imbalance in electrical charge. Free radicals seek to achieve balance by stealing electrons from other molecules. If they grab electrons from neurons, the brain cells typically suffer DNA or other cellular damage but don't die. Damage to neural DNA, if widespread, has been linked to a host of brain disorders, including dementia.

Antioxidants act like an open bank vault offering free electrons for the roving antioxidants. Free radicals steal ample and easily available electrons from antioxidants in the bloodstream instead of targeting neural tissues. Good sources of antioxidants include blueberries, blackberries, cranberries, and other complex berries; walnuts; artichokes; and coffee.

▶ **Restricting the intake of sugar.** Especially try to skip the refined kind, found abundantly in widely advertised sugary drinks, as well as in cookies and cakes.

▶ **Eating the right kinds of carbohydrates.** Fruits, vegetables, and whole grains—as opposed to the processed grain flour of many commercially baked breads—provide carbohydrates and fiber without excess calories. Fiber helps the body regulate blood sugar levels and reduces cravings for fattier foods.

▶ **Drinking very moderate amounts of caffeine and alcohol.** Caffeine, found in coffee, cocoa, tea, cola, and chocolate, stimulates the brain. Americans consume about 200 milligrams a day, or roughly the equivalent of about one to two cups of coffee. Caffeine works by blocking the neurotransmitter adenosine, which induces sedation and eases pain and anxiety. By dampening adenosine, caffeine not only encourages the jitters but also raises a sense of alertness by arousing the cerebral cortex. In small amounts, such as two cups of coffee or less taken in the morning, caffeine accelerates thinking, boosts energy levels, and briefly increases physical performance. It may even lower depression enough to lessen suicide levels. Too much caffeine, however, raises stress and blood pressure levels and interferes with sleep, which the brain needs to rejuvenate itself.

Likewise, a little bit of alcohol, such as one glass once in a while in the evening, has been shown to have health benefits, but alcohol is toxic to brain functions—hence the origin of the word *intoxication*. More than a little bit in the short run interferes with basic cognitive functions, such as memory, by blocking neural firing and the flow of oxygen, and in the long run can shrink the brain and also damage the liver in ways that affect mood, sleep, and attention span. Yet, alcohol in small amounts is believed to encourage the body to reduce the concentration of bad forms of cholesterol in the bloodstream. If you're going to drink alcohol, try limiting yourself to a glass of red wine with dinner. Red wine contains resveratrol, an antioxidant and anti-inflammatory chemical.

▶ **Drinking plenty of water.** The brain is 80 percent water, and it needs to stay wet. Dehydration impairs mental function, and in extreme cases, can cause a person to

BE MINDFUL OF YOUR CAFFEINE

A little caffeine boost goes a long way

How much caffeine do you use each day? Caffeine is a stimulant, which in modest amounts can boost alertness and enhance learning and memory. However, too much caffeine can have the opposite effect, lowering memory performance as it leaves us jittery and unable to focus and learn.

➲ CAFFEINE SOURCES in our diet include coffee, black or green tea, caffeinated sodas, and chocolate. The recent popularity of energy drinks and caffeine as an additive has made us all more vulnerable to getting higher doses of caffeine in our diet than we might have intended.

➲ CAFFEINE AFFECTS each of us differently. Spend some time this week figuring out where you get your caffeine (don't forget the chocolate!), and how to best balance your use of it.

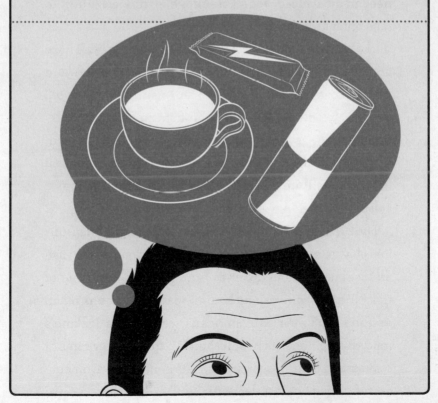

hallucinate or even die. Ohio University researchers found that mental functions become compromised long before dehydration becomes severe. They subjected healthy men and women in their 60s to tests of brain functions, including examinations of memory, eye-hand coordination, and attention. They also gathered data on test subjects' hydration levels. Those whose bodies contained a proper amount of water posted significantly higher scores on the cognitive tests.

▶ **Swallowing a daily multivitamin and mineral supplement.** B-complex vitamins are crucial for brain health, and although you likely will get all the vitamins you need in a balanced, vegetable-rich diet, it doesn't hurt to take out a little dietary insurance.

▶ **Taking omega-3 fatty acids regularly.** These acids, also called DHA (docosahexaenoic acid) and EPA (eicosapentaenoic acid), occur naturally in fish oil; you can get them by eating the fish themselves, or by taking them as pill supplements containing 500 milligrams of DHA and EPA. Vegetarians can skip the fish oil and substitute flaxseed oil, either in pill form or as a salad dressing.

The brain draws upon these fatty acids to grow neurons and elevate mood. Evidence of the link between eating fish and feeling contented comes from Iceland. Residents of that North Atlantic island country eat five times as much seafood each year as Americans, yet despite Iceland's long, dark winters, its people suffer extremely low rates of depression. Some research suggests benefits from omega-3s in fighting against dementia.

....

Eat Less, Live Longer

The benefits of a moderate diet have been known for centuries

In middle age, Venetian nobleman Alvise "Luigi" Cornaro faced the prospect of an early death because of his poor health. He examined his life and blamed his gluttony and hedonistic lifestyle. So, on his doctor's advice, he set about making changes.

Cornaro reduced his diet to bread, eggs in broth, a little meat, and new wine. His health returned so completely that he lived to be 98, dying in 1566.

When Cornaro was 83, friends urged him to record his story, not only because he had lived so long, but also because he maintained mental clarity. Cornaro's book, *Discorsi della Vita Sobria (Discourses on the Sober Life)*, became a Renaissance best seller all over Europe, not only in his own day but also in the years that followed. Printers produced dozens of editions in England in the 18th and 19th centuries, and the book still goes through reprints in the United States.

Readers found much common sense in Cornaro's cardinal rule of temperance: "Whosoever wishes to eat much must eat little," meaning that abstaining from gluttony promotes longevity. Modern science has added its own voice in support of Cornaro's enthusiasm for eating less with studies linking severely reduced caloric intake to greater longevity in rats.

....

▶ JUMP-START YOUR ROUTINE
Staying active is key to brain health

....

Regular exercise is good not only for the heart and muscles, but also for the brain. Movement of arms, legs, trunk, and head occurs because of coordinated firing of neural networks in the brain's motor cortex, cerebellum, and other regions. And anything that increases blood flow to the brain, such as a heart-stimulating run or weight lifting in the gym, improves every brain function because all neurons devour oxygen. Other brain benefits of exercise include greater control of blood sugar levels, which damage blood vessels in the brain when they're too high, and stronger heart muscle to pump blood more efficiently. And, of course, vigorous exercise encourages deep, natural sleep.

Physical exercise has also been linked to the growth of new cells, blood vessels, and neural connections in the brain. It boosts mood, so much so that doctors often prescribe exercise as part of the therapy for patients with depression. And it guards against brain shrinkage among the elderly.

The scientific studies that back up those conclusions are growing and becoming more expansive every day. A study of 1,740 people by the Group Health Cooperative in Seattle found that those in the group who did some form of exercise at least three times a week cut their risk for dementia by 38 percent compared to their sedentary peers. A Hawaiian study of more than 2,220 Japanese Americans age 71 and older revealed that those who exercised the most over a six-year period halved their risk of developing dementia. A 1994 Harvard study concluded that men who burned more than 2,500 calories a day in aerobic exercise were substantially less likely to develop clinical depression than men who were less active. And in another study, published in 2007 by a University of Illinois research team, physically fit third and fifth graders at four elementary schools academically outperformed their peers who were not physically fit. Those results, found in examining 239 children, held true regardless of the pupils' race, sex, or socioeconomic background.

Pump It Up

Good forms of physical exercise include ones that work your heart and lungs, as well as those that make your large muscle tissues burn with exertion. Aerobic exercise, such as jogging or swimming, gets the heart pumping and growing stronger. But weight-bearing exercises, such as pumping iron at the gym, also are important, and particularly so as the body and brain grow older. Greater strength and flexibility in the limbs and trunk, along with improved balance, help prevent the devastating falls common with the elderly.

GET PHYSICAL!

Simple aerobic exercise does wonders for your brain

BRAIN BOOSTER

It's time to try one of the most "tried-and-true" things you can do to boost your brain's well-being—aerobic exercise. Recent research shows that regular aerobic exercise can:

➡ IMPROVE your memory and other skills, such as attention, processing speed, and executive control, which matter to daily intellectual performance.

➡ SIGNIFICANTLY DECREASE your risk for dementia.

➡ SIGNIFICANTLY REDUCE your risk for or be an important part of managing medical conditions, such as obesity, diabetes, and hypertension.

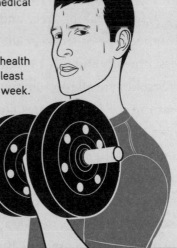

Start today on the road to better brain health by boosting your exercise time. Get at least 30 minutes of exercise several days a week. Even brisk walking is beneficial to brain health. Make it easier to stick with your exercise plan by penciling in time to work out, finding an exercise buddy, or setting clear exercise goals with built-in rewards.

The best workout for you is one that you'll enjoy doing again and again, because it has to be part of a continuing routine. The exercise should challenge your body, but not pose a threat to it. And it should challenge your brain; new forms of exercise, or new twists on old ones, provide the novelty that helps foster and strengthen neural connections.

▶ SAFETY FIRST
Recognizing the risk of stroke

It's not enough to eat well and exercise. Keeping your brain healthy requires that you keep it safe from injury. Two of the most common brain hazards are stroke and concussion.

Stroke suddenly restricts blood flow in the vessels leading to the brain, or in the brain itself. When brain cells are cut off from the oxygen in red blood cells, they die in a few minutes. Ischemic strokes involve blockage of blood vessels servicing a particular part of the brain. This can occur through formation of a blood clot in the brain, or by a clot traveling to the brain after forming in another part of the body, breaking free, and traveling through the bloodstream. Another type of stroke, called hemorrhagic, occurs when a blood vessel breaks and fills a brain region with blood.

Strokes are all too common. They are the fourth leading cause of death in the United States and the primary cause of disability. The types of brain damage caused by localized strokes depend upon the function of the affected neural networks. Strokes in the motor control regions restrict motion. Strokes in language-processing regions affect production and understanding of speech and writing. Strokes can also affect memory, mood, analytical abilities, and other cognitive functions. In vital areas such as the brain stem, they can swiftly kill.

IS IT A STROKE?

This simple test can help you detect the warning signs

Stroke is a major cause of brain injury, the leading cause of adult disability, and the fourth leading cause of death in the United States. Recently, there have been tremendous advances in our ability to both prevent and treat for stroke. But you have to know what to look for and be ready to act quickly. I find that few folks really know the signs of a stroke—so let's learn them! This simple three-step test, developed by researchers, is highly effective in identifying a stroke. If you suspect that someone you know is having a stroke, try the following three things. If the person fails any of them, get to the ER as quickly as possible for an evaluation:

➡ **STEP 1: SMILE**
Ask the person to smile. Look for asymmetry (unevenness) in his or her expression. (For example, check to see if one corner of the mouth droops.)

➡ **STEP 2: RAISE BOTH ARMS**
Ask the person to raise both arms. Look for asymmetry in the height of the hands.

➡ **STEP 3: REPEAT A SIMPLE SENTENCE**
Ask the person to repeat a simple sentence, such as "No ifs, ands, or buts." Check for slurring or other disruption of speech.

Want to know more? Visit the National Stroke Association's website at *www.stroke.org*.

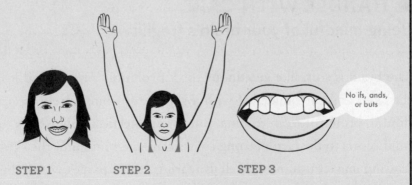

No ifs, ands, or buts

STEP 1   STEP 2   STEP 3

A Swift Response Can Save a Life

Ischemic strokes usually respond well to treatment if it is given within three hours of suffering an attack. Administration of a drug called tPA, for tissue plasminogen activator, can help save brain tissue within that three-hour window. (Hemorrhagic strokes, on the other hand, might be made worse by tPA; doctors need to establish the kind of stroke before treatment.) For ischemic strokes, it's important to recognize stroke risk factors and indicators of stroke's onset to get treatment within that 180-minute window. Quicker response is even better. According to a study published in 2010 in the British journal *Lancet,* patients given blood-thinning tPA within 90 minutes of a stroke were more than twice as likely to have a good recovery than those who did not receive the medication.

The highest risk factors for strokes are those that promote disorders in the blood vessels. These include high blood pressure, high cholesterol, hardening of the arteries, diabetes, and smoking, all of which restrict the flow of red blood cells. Warning signs commonly include sudden muscle or mental impairment, such as confusion, numbness, paralysis, and sudden headache.

▶ HANDLE WITH CARE
Being mindful of your brain's fragility

The brain is soft, like gelatinous tofu. Evolution has encased it in the skull and surrounded it with a shock-absorbing cerebrospinal fluid to protect it from trauma. But that protection only works for mild blows to the head. Strong blows slam the brain into the skull, causing impact trauma as well as tearing neural tissues where they bash into ridges on the underside of the skull's bony plates. Not

CHECK YOUR BLOOD PRESSURE

Learn your numbers and reduce your risk of stroke

This tip comes right out of the medical textbooks: Take a few minutes today to check your blood pressure.

➡ **REDUCING YOUR RISK**

Hypertension, or high blood pressure, when not controlled by lifestyle or medication, can seriously increase your risk for stroke, which in turn can cause disability, memory loss, or death.

You can have your blood pressure checked at most pharmacies, many of which have a blood pressure machine available. If your pressure seems higher than usual, follow up with your doctor. Hypertension can readily be managed.

Want to reduce your risk for stroke? A 2008 study from the Harvard School of Public Health found that people could reduce their risk for stroke by up to 80 percent by leading a brain-healthy lifestyle, including regular exercise, a healthy diet, maintaining a healthy weight, and not smoking.

Now that's something to think about!

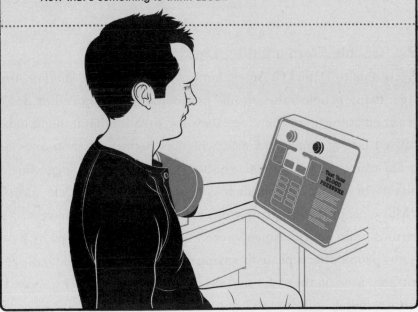

every impact or concussion causes lasting injury; variations in the power of the blow and its location, as well as the genetics of the concussion sufferer, lead to unpredictable outcomes.

Concussion is a brain injury that can have short- and long-term effects ranging from dizziness to serious cognitive impairment. Concussions frequently occur to soldiers and athletes in sports where collisions are considered part of the game. Boxing and football probably come to mind as the most likely sources of concussion, but serious brain injuries can also occur in soccer, basketball, baseball, and other less brutal sports. For example, researchers at the University of Cincinnati found reduced amounts of gray matter in the brains of college soccer players compared with peers who did not play the game. They linked the damage to blows to the head, including the act of heading a ball in flight to redirect it toward the goal or another player. Falls in noncontact sports also can cause concussions.

Big Trouble From a Little Bump

According to Daniel G. Amen, author of *Magnificent Mind at Any Age,* many people suffer a mild traumatic brain injury but don't realize it at the time. Therefore, they don't realize that it might have caused lasting damage. Amen, who has performed thousands of brain scans, is quick to notice patterns of brain injury suggesting a history of impact trauma, such as concussions from violent sports. "Many people forget or they did not realize that they have had a serious brain injury," Amen wrote. "You would be amazed by how many people after repeatedly saying no to this question suddenly get an 'aha' look on their face and say, 'Why yes, I fell out of a second-story window at age seven.' "

BRAIN INSIGHT

The NFL's Concussion Crisis

Professional football players are on the front lines of head injuries

Jim McMahon won a Super Bowl as quarterback of the 1985 Chicago Bears. Time and again in his career, McMahon bounced back from injuries, including bruised ribs, a lacerated kidney, a sore neck, bumps and bruises incurred by sliding headfirst to gain extra yards, and chronic concussions.

Today, McMahon is one of the highest profile litigants accusing the NFL of hiding vital information about concussions in order to keep players in the game. "We knew there was going to be a chance for injury," McMahon told ESPN. "But we didn't know about the head trauma. And they did, and that's the whole reason for this lawsuit."

Concussion occurs when a sudden jerk rams the brain into the skull, damaging brain tissue. Immediate effects may include dizziness, imbalance, and unconsciousness. Long-term effects vary greatly, but may include confusion, memory loss, depression, and suicidal thoughts. McMahon has trouble forming memories. Junior Seau, a former San Diego Chargers linebacker who took his life in 2012, suffered many concussions.

In 2011, the NFL changed its rules to better protect players showing signs of brain trauma. But it was too late to protect itself against scores of complaints that were consolidated into one big lawsuit against pro football in 2012.

Amen notes that suffering a head injury increases later incidence of drug abuse, alcoholism, mood disorders, and other behavioral changes. This might be expected for damage to the frontal lobes, where the brain executes control over instinctive actions associated with the older and deeper portions of the mammalian brain. If a concussion weakens the brain's ability to reason, make good decisions, or override the circuitry that regulates pleasure seeking in favor of long-term benefits, it's no wonder that chronic concussion sufferers often exhibit self-destructive behaviors. Two high-profile cases in spring 2012 were the suicides of former NFL players Junior Seau and Ray Easterling, both of whom suffered brain trauma from playing the game.

BRAIN INSIGHT

Automatic Reboot

Brain cells can make new pathways when the old ones are lost

Brain cells die when deprived of oxygen by a stroke. When those affected neural circuits play a key role in moving an arm or leg, the stroke patient loses some or all control of that limb.

However, brains can rewire themselves to regain lost movement. Psychologist Edward Taub of the University of Alabama at Birmingham has gotten impressive results restoring movement by enrolling stroke patients in "constraint induced movement therapy." He has stroke patients selectively try to use their affected arm or leg while deliberately avoiding use of their unaffected partners. Taub found that, in just two weeks, the patients' neural circuitry had rewired itself, a process known as cortical reorganization, to bypass dead neural arrays. Professional musicians who had lost some control of their arms were able to return to work.

The mere act of thinking about moving a stroke-affected limb can help rewire the brain. Researchers at the Drake Center/University of Cincinnati put subjects affected by stroke through visualization exercises that included listening to a CD while mentally orchestrating physical therapy exercises. Even years after a stroke, patients who added the visualization exercises to their therapy routines found greater improvement than those who did the physical therapy alone.

Amen's advice is to teach children about the importance of the brain and insist that they take pains to protect it. Sports enthusiasts

PROTECT YOUR NOGGIN

Simple precautions can help to keep your brain from harm

Head injury, especially repeated head injury or concussion, can also mean brain injury. Recovery from such damage can take months, with symptoms including difficulty concentrating, double vision, and light sensitivity.

Even those of us who spend more time watching football than playing it can take steps to protect our heads. Here are some easy tips for taking care of your precious brain day in and day out:

➡ **WEAR A HELMET**
Everyone should wear a helmet when participating in a sport that carries a risk of head injury. Your helmet should fit snugly and comfortably, and should be strapped.

➡ **WEAR SEAT BELTS**
Wearing a seat belt is essential to restraining your head and the rest of your body in case of a car accident. In most states, it's also the law.

➡ **AVOID RISK**
Use your noggin to protect your head. Be thoughtful about what might increase your risk for a head injury: Look for tripping hazards on the floor or poor lighting in stairways.

➡ **IN THE EVENT OF A CONCUSSION, GET EVALUATED AND TREATED**
If you or a loved one suffers a concussion, see your doctor and follow his or her recommendations.

Want more information on concussion? Visit the Centers for Disease Control website at *www.cdc.gov/concussion* to learn more.

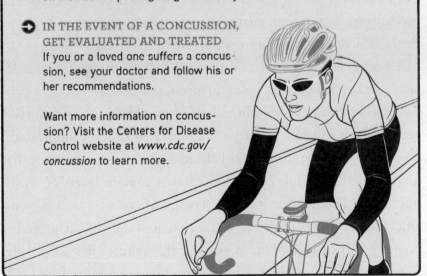

might choose competition with low levels of risk, or wear protective headgear before engaging in higher levels of risk. Helmets for bicyclists and motorcyclists are a must. So, too, are the right kinds of helmets for football players.

The Hazards of High Impact

Football players as young as third graders experience blows to the head that would be considered high magnitude for college players, according to studies by biomedical engineering professor Stefan Duma of the Virginia Tech University College of Engineering. Duma and his team of researchers provided helmets equipped with impact sensors to seven- and eight-year-old players and collected data on more than 750 blows to the boys' heads that occurred during games and practice. The most severe blow registered 100 Gs, or gravitational forces. One of the most surprising discoveries was that most of the worst blows to the head occurred during practice and not during the emotionally heightened contact of actual games. New kinds of impact sensors include high-tech mouth guards that record the severity of blows to the head and relay that information wirelessly to the sidelines.

Duma aims to take what he has learned from the studies to redesign football helmets to make them safer. Virginia Tech also published safety ratings for 15 brands of football helmets, with several receiving top-end endorsements and one rated "not recommended." The key to creating an effective helmet is physics. Most helmets that are designed to handle high-impact blows contain layers of crushable foam. The foam absorbs the energy of collision as it flattens, shielding the brain from the worst potential damage. It probably comes as no surprise that, in general, the helmets that afford the most protection have higher price tags.

But isn't the brain worth the extra protection? Pinching pennies is a poor strategy for ensuring long-term brain health. If you do all you can to protect and nurture your brain, from eating and exercising right to shielding it from injury, you will give yourself the best odds of enjoying a long and brain-healthy life.

BRAIN INSIGHT

Fast-Forward

Will brain-computer partnerships be the norm one hundred years from now?

Physicist Michio Kaku, extrapolating into the future, has plotted the acceleration of technology and devised a scenario of life in 2100, when computers and the human brain will communicate directly with one another.

As described in Kaku's book *Physics of the Future*, it's a sometimes dizzying world of starships, Martian colonies, and DNA manipulation. In daily life, computer–brain interfaces make life more comfortable, as he outlines in a description of a typical day.

In the morning, you telepathically tell servant computers to adjust room temperature, prepare breakfast, and play music. You insert Internet-display contact lenses and scan the news without ever having to hold a digital pad, much less a newspaper.

At the office, brains telepathically control robots doing difficult work—in Kaku's scenario, underwater construction.

Back home, you ask your computer assistant to help you shop. Your brain–computer interface calls up images of stores and goods, and you make your choices. You could buy online, but instead you telepathically summon your car to go to the mall.

The scenario progresses through dating, marriage, and parenthood. Along the way, you make choices. Then, as now, in Kaku's vision, you can always choose, including decisions about health and offspring. Brain never becomes slave to machine.

GLOSSARY

....

AGNOSIA. The inability to interpret sensory impressions.

ALZHEIMER'S DISEASE. The most common cause of dementia, primarily affecting memory, thinking, and reasoning.

AMYGDALA. Structure in the brain's limbic system that plays an important role in emotional learning.

ANTIOXIDANT. Nutrient or chemical such as beta-carotene or vitamin C. Inhibits oxidation and may protect cells from damage caused by free radicals.

APHASIA. Neurodegenerative condition affecting the ability to understand or express language, generally as a result of stroke or similar brain trauma.

AUTONOMIC NERVOUS SYSTEM. The division of the peripheral nervous system that controls cardiac muscles, smooth muscles, and glands.

AXON. The hairlike extension of a neuron that sends out impulses.

BRAIN STEM. The portion of the brain just above the spinal cord, consisting of the midbrain, pons, and medulla.

CENTRAL NERVOUS SYSTEM. The brain and spinal cord.

CEREBELLUM. Part of the brain behind the medulla and pons; governs coordinated muscle activity.

CEREBRAL CORTEX. Outer layer of the cerebral hemispheres, responsible for conscious experience, thought, and planning.

CEREBRUM. The two cerebral hemispheres that make up most of the brain.

CORTISOL. A hormone released by the adrenal cortex in periods of extended stress.

DELIRIUM. Temporary mental disturbance marked by hallucinations, disorganized speech, and confusion.

DEMENTIA. A progressive mental condition, such as Alzheimer's disease, characterized by the development of many cognitive defects, such as disorientation and the inability to remember family members or make coherent plans.

DENDRITE. The branching extension of the neuron cell body that receives electrical signals.

DIENCEPHALON. Part of the forebrain that includes the thalamus, hypothalamus, and epithalamus.

FOREBRAIN. The forward portion of the brain, including the regions associated with cognition.

FREE RADICALS. Atoms or groups of atoms with an odd number of electrons. Free radicals can start a chemical chain reaction within cells that can damage their DNA or other structures.

FRONTAL LOBE. One of four lobes in the front of the cerebral cortex responsible for movement and planning.

GANGLIA (*SINGULAR, GANGLION*). Groups of nerve cell bodies outside of the central nervous system.

HIPPOCAMPUS. Seahorse-shaped structure in the brain's limbic system that is involved in learning, memory, and emotion.

HYPOTHALAMUS. Structure in the brain's diencephalon that monitors the autonomic nervous system.

INSULA. Region of the cerebral cortex linked to emotion and awareness of body states.

LIFE EXPECTANCY. Expected number of years of life based on statistical probability that can be measured from birth or from any other age.

LIMBIC SYSTEM. Deep-brain structure containing various structures involved in emotions and behavior.

LONGEVITY. The length of life.

MEDULLA OBLONGATA. The lowest part of the brain stem.

MENINGES. Protective coverings of the brain and spinal cord.

METHOD OF LOCI. A memory technique in which items to be remembered are associated with locations.

MIDBRAIN. The brain stem between the pons and diencephalon.

MOTOR NEURON. Nerve that carries impulses from the brain and spinal cord to effectors, either muscles or glands.

MYELIN SHEATH. The multilayered fatty covering that insulates most nerve fibers.

MYOPIA. A condition in which images focus in front of the eye's retina, resulting in nearsightedness.

NEUROGLIA. Cells of the nervous system that support and protect neurons; also called glial cells.

NEURON. A nerve cell.

NEUROTRANSMITTER. Chemical released by a neuron at a synapse.

OPTOGENETICS. A technology that allows users to control living systems using light.

PARASYMPATHETIC DIVISION. Subdivision of the autonomic nervous system responsible for overseeing the conservation and restoration of the body's energy.

PARIETAL LOBE. A middle portion of each cerebral hemisphere that processes bodily sensations.

PERIPHERAL NERVOUS SYSTEM. The portion of the nervous system, consisting of nerves and ganglia, that lies outside the brain.

PONS. The bridge-like part of the brain stem between the medulla and midbrain.

PREFRONTAL CORTEX. Brain region located in the anterior frontal lobe, responsible for reasoning, planning, empathy, and abstract ideas.

PRESBYCUSIS. Age-related hearing loss resulting from degenerative changes in the ear.

PRESBYOPIA. Age-related changes in vision that lead to an inability to focus on close objects.

PROPRIOCEPTION. The perception of the position of the body in space.

RECEPTOR. Specialized cell or portion of a nerve cell that responds to sensory input and converts it to an electrical signal.

SENSORY NEURON. Nerve cell that carries sensory information into the brain and spinal cord.

SOMATIC NERVOUS SYSTEM. The division of the peripheral nervous system that activates skeletal muscles.

SPINAL CORD. The bundle of nervous tissue that runs down the center of the vertebral column, carrying messages to and from the brain.

SYMPATHETIC DIVISION. The subdivision of the autonomic nervous system responsible for overseeing activation of body systems in response to stress.

SYNAPSE. The junction between two neurons or between a neuron and an effector, such as a gland or muscle.

SYNESTHESIA. A condition in which the stimulation of one sense is simultaneously perceived by another sense or senses.

TEMPORAL LOBE. A portion of the cerebral cortex, below the Sylvian fissure, that processes speech and memory.

THALAMUS. A structure made of two egg-shaped masses of gray matter in the brain; acts as a relay station for sensory information flowing into the brain.

VENTRICLES. Large interior spaces in the forebrain and brain stem filled with cerebrospinal fluid.

VESTIBULAR SYSTEM. The portion of the inner ear responsible for balance and posture.

FURTHER READING

Amen, Daniel G. *Magnificent Mind at Any Age: Natural Ways to Unleash Your Brain's Maximum Potential.* New York: Three Rivers Press, 2008.

Begley, Sharon. *Train Your Mind, Change Your Brain: How a New Science Reveals Our Extraordinary Potential to Transform Ourselves.* New York: Ballantine Books, 2007.

Butler, Gillian, and Tony Hope. *Managing Your Mind: The Mental Fitness Guide,* 2nd ed. New York: Oxford University Press, 2007.

Cohen, Gene D. *The Creative Age: Awakening Human Potential in the Second Half of Life.* New York: Avon Books, 2000.

Eagleman, David. *Incognito: The Secret Lives of the Brain.* New York: Canongate, 2011.

Foer, Joshua. *Moonwalking With Einstein: The Art and Science of Remembering Everything.* New York: Penguin Press, 2011.

Gottschall, Jonathan. *The Storytelling Animal: How Stories Make Us Human.* Boston: Houghton Mifflin Harcourt, 2012.

Green, Cynthia R., and Joan Beloff. *Through the Seasons: An Activity Book for Memory-Challenged Adults and Caregivers.* Baltimore, Md.: Johns Hopkins University Press, 2008.

Green, Cynthia R., and the editors of *Prevention. Brainpower Game Plan: Foods, Moves, and Games to Clear Brain Fog, Boost Memory, and Age-Proof Your Mind in 4 Weeks!* Emmaus, Pa.: Rodale, 2009.

Green, Cynthia R. *30 Days to Total Brain Health: A Whole Month's Worth of Daily Tips to Boost Your Memory and Build Better Brain Power.* Upper Montclair, N.J.: Memory Arts, 2011.

Green, Cynthia R. *The Total Memory Workout: 8 Easy Steps to Maximum Memory Fitness.* New York: Bantam Books, 1999.

Hanson, Rick, with Richard Mendius. *Buddha's Brain: The Practical Neuroscience of Happiness, Love and Wisdom*. Oakland, Calif.: New Harbinger Publications, 2009.

Hayflick, Leonard. *How and Why We Age*. New York: Ballantine Books, 1994.

Higbee, Kenneth L. *Your Memory: How It Works and How to Improve It*. New York: Marlowe and Company, 1996.

Horstman, Judith. *The Scientific American Healthy Aging Brain: The Neuroscience of Making the Most of Your Mature Mind*. San Francisco: Jossey-Bass, 2012.

Johnson, Steven. *Everything Bad Is Good for You: How Today's Popular Culture is Actually Making Us Smarter*. New York: Riverhead Books, 2005.

Kaku, Michio. *Physics of the Future: How Science Will Shape Human Destiny and Our Daily Lives by the Year 2100*. New York: Doubleday, 2011.

Katz, Lawrence C. and Manning Rubin. *Keep Your Brain Alive: 83 Neurobic Exercises to Help Prevent Memory Loss and Increase Mental Fitness*. New York: Workman Press, 1999.

Kurzweil, Ray. *The Singularity Is Near: When Humans Transcend Biology*. New York: Viking, 2005.

Michelon, Pascale. *Max Your Memory: The Complete Visual Program*. New York: DK Publishing, 2012.

Nordstrom, Nancy Merz. *Learning Later, Living Greater: The Secret for Making the Most of Your After-50 Years*. Boulder, Colo.: Sentient Publications, 2006.

Ramachandran, V. S. *The Tell-Tale Brain: A Neuroscientist's Quest for What Makes Us Human*. New York: W. W. Norton, 2011.

Ratey, John. *A User's Guide to the Brain: Perception, Attention, and the Four Theaters of the Brain*. New York: Random House, 2001.

Restak, Richard. *Mozart's Brain and the Fighter Pilot: Unleashing Your Brain's Potential*. New York: Harmony Books, 2001.

Restak, Richard. *Older and Wiser: How to Maintain Peak Mental Ability for as Long as You Live*. New York: Simon & Schuster, 1997.

Restak, Richard. *Poe's Heart and the Mountain Climber: Exploring the Effect of Anxiety on Our Brains and Our Culture*. New York: Harmony Books, 2004.

Rowe, John W., and Robert L. Kahn. *Successful Aging: The MacArthur Foundation Study*. New York: Pantheon Books, 1998.

Schacter, Daniel L. *The Seven Sins of Memory: How the Mind Forgets and Remembers*. Boston: Houghton Mifflin, 2001.

Schwartz, Jeffrey M., and Sharon Begley. *The Mind and the Brain: Neuroplasticity and the Power of Mental Force*. New York: Regan Books/HarperCollins, 2002.

Snowdon, David. *Aging With Grace: What the Nun Study Teaches Us About Leading Longer, Healthier, and More Meaningful Lives*. New York: Bantam Books, 2001.

Sweeney, Michael S. *Brain: The Complete Mind: How It Develops, How It Works, and How to Keep It Sharp*. Washington, D.C.: National Geographic Press, 2009.

ABOUT THE AUTHOR

Michael S. Sweeney is a professor in the E. W. Scripps School of Journalism at Ohio University, where he heads the graduate program and teaches classes in reporting, writing, and editing. He has written several books for National Geographic, including *Brain: The Complete Mind* and *God Grew Tired of Us*. He lives in Athens, Ohio, with his wife, Carolyn.

ABOUT THE CONSULTANT

Cynthia R. Green, Ph.D., is a clinical psychologist, author, and leading expert on memory wellness and brain health. An assistant clinical professor of psychiatry at the Mount Sinai School of Medicine in New York, Dr. Green provides training, consultation, and keynote services on all things brain health to individuals, companies, and organizations through Memory Arts, LLC, and the Total Brain Health program *(www.totalbrain health.com)*. Dr. Green appears frequently in the media as a contributor on brain wellness. A graduate of Smith College and New York University, Dr. Green lives with her family in New Jersey.

INDEX

A

Acetylcholine 13
ACTIVE (Advanced Cognitive
    Training for Independent
    and Vital Elderly) 151
Adderall (attention-enhancing
    drug) 117
Adenosine 210
Adolescents 25, 202
Adrenaline 36, 166
Advanced Cognitive Training
    for Independent and Vital
    Elderly (ACTIVE) 151
Aerobic exercise 33, 215
Affection, for stress 168, 173
Aging
    balance 77–78
    brain decline 26, 38
    conjunctive searches 113
    depression 177–179
    hearing loss 56, 58, 228
    information processing
        speed 26
    language processing 85–87,
        96–97
    memory 26, 141–142,
        145–150
    motor skills 68
    neurons 26, 38
    neurotransmitters 179
    plasticity 8, 26–27
    senses 26, 43–44, 48, 59
    sleep disturbances 179
    tip-of-the-tongue experiences
        85–87
    vision 48, 50–52
    visual attention 113
Agnosia 104–105, 226
Air traffic control 184–185
Albert, Marilyn 159
Alcohol
    abuse 34, 68
    and loss of balance 68
    moderation 206, 209–210
Alzheimer, Alois 149
Alzheimer's 149
    avoiding effects 40
    in bilinguals 101
    checklist 146–147
    and cognitive reserve 40
    definition 226
    early indicators 146–147, 157
    medications 157
    memory 146–147
    prevalence 149
    prevention efforts 153–154

risk factors 154–155
    stages 149
Amen, Daniel G. 17, 220–222
Ames, Adelbert, Jr. 108
Ames room 107, 108
Amputations 112
Amygdala 124, 226
Anderson, G. John 48
Antidepressants 174
Antioxidants 56, 68, 155, 209,
    226
Anxiety see Stress
Aphasia 226
Athletes
    altered perception 108–109
    concussion 218, 220–225
Attention 104–119
    Brain Boosters 106, 111,
        114, 116, 118
    cognitive fitness 37
    drowning out distractions
        112–113, 115, 117–119
    executive function 98
    exercise for 32
    illusions 107–109
    selective attention 112–113,
        115, 117–119
    vision therapy 110, 112
Attention-deficit disorder 117
Attentional blink 115
Autism 22
Autism spectrum disorder 135
Autonomic nervous system 226
Axons 10–12, 22, 66, 226

B

Bach-y-Rita, Paul 63
Backward walking 79
Balance 74–83
    aging 77–78
    coordinated by cerebellum
        20–21
    dominant/nondominant
        sides 31
    dynamic balance 77
    exercises for 79–83
    loss of 78
    motion circuits 66, 68
    and muscle coordination 65
    static balance 77
    testing 80–81
    vestibular system 74–75, 77,
        79, 229
Basal ganglia 66
Beeman, Mark 189
Beethoven, Ludwig van 181

Begley, Sharon 176–177
Bell, Alexander Graham 100
Bell, Gordon 140, 141
Berkeley, George 42–43
Berman, Marc 32
Beta-amyloid plaques 149
Bhattacharya, Joydeep 188–189
Bialystok, Ellen 98, 100, 101
Bilingualism 98–103
Blindness 63
Blood pressure 219
Body fat 207
Body functions, regulation 19
Bradley, Scott 54–55
Brain
    anatomy 14, 16–18
    parts 14
    percentage used 23
    prenatal development 21–22
    structure 10
    weight 38
    see also Attention; Brain
        health; Controlling your
        brain; Language; Living
        smart; Memory; Mood
        and creativity; Movement;
        Senses; Sustain your brain
Brain Boosters
    aerobic exercise 215
    balance 31
    beat the clock 118
    brain game night 187
    breathe like a lion 176
    caffeine moderation 211
    calendar use (memory) 143
    categories (memory) 139
    chunking (memory tech-
        nique) 130
    coloring 165
    driving skills 53
    eye opener 47
    focus 50
    goals 27
    haiku 94
    honorable opposition 199
    hug five 168
    jigsaw puzzles 111
    juggling 76
    learn a new language 99
    listing ways your brain is
        great 163
    make a match (memory) 127
    make a movie (memory and
        attention) 136
    map reading 114
    masking tape usage 192

meditation 171
memory connection tech-
  nique 122
mindfulness 190
olfactory memory 57
online games 61
origami 39
poetry memorization 156
protect your head 223
reach out and reconnect 175
repetition (memory booster)
  152
reverse perceptions (mir-
  rors) 49
school memories 144
see squared (perception)
  106
sentence scramble 86
small steps 15
stretch at your desk 69
tap a tune 67
ten steps to brain health 24
touch exercise 62
vocabulary 93
walking backward 79
wear your watch upside
  down 35
what's in the clouds 201
word search game 89
write a love song 180
X marks the spot 116
yoga 73
yoga breathing 176
Brain chemistry 13, 36–37
Brain health 28–41
  body fitness 30, 32–34, 36
  Brain Boosters 31, 35, 39
  butterfly effect 29–30
  cognitive fitness 37–41,
    150–151, 153
  vitality 36–37
Brain injuries 25, 95, 218,
  220–225
Brain-machine interfaces 225
Brain stem 21, 66, 164, 226
BrainPort 63
Breakfast 205
Breathing 21, 172, 176
Broca's area 88
Buddha's Brain (Hanson) 161,
  182
Burke, Deborah 87, 89, 91
Butler, Gillian 198
Butterfly effect 29–30

C
Caffeine 34, 209–210, 211
Calendar use 143
Carbohydrates 209
Central nervous system 226
Cerebellum 20–21, 25, 66,
  68, 226

Cerebral cortex
  Alzheimer's 149
  arousal through caffeine 210
  definition 226
  development 21
  functions 14
  growth 7
Cerebrum 14, 16, 66, 226
Champollion, Jean-François 88
Chang San-Feng 80
Chaos theory 29–30
Chase, William G. 129
Chemistry *see* Brain chemistry
Children
  bilingualism 98, 101–102
  high-stress environments 36
Chunking (memory technique)
  126, 128–130
Cicero, Marcus Tullius 131–
  132, 138
Clinical depression *see* Depression
Cloud-viewing 201
Cochlea 52, 54
Cochlear implants 54
Cognitive behavioral therapy
  174, 176–177
Cognitive fitness 37–41, 150–
  151, 153
Cognitive reserve 38, 40
Cognitive therapy 195–198
Cohen, Gene D. 179
Coloring 165
Communication 167
Computers
  communicating with human
    brain 225
  driving-skills programs
    118–119
  and myopia 44
Concussion 218, 220–225
Conjunctive searches 113
Constraint induced movement
  therapy 222
Controlling your brain 184–203
  Brian Boosters 187, 190,
    192, 199, 201
  coping with stimuli 186–191
  making decisions 185–186,
    191
  memories and mood 200–203
  positive attitude 193,
    195–198
  taking control 191–195
Cooper, Bradley 23
Cornaro, Alvise "Luigi" 213
Corpus callosum 14
Cortisol (stress hormone) 36,
  166, 169, 226
Creativity 165, 179–183

D
Dance 158–159

Davidson, Lisa 101–102
Daviglus, Martha L. 153
Daydreams 162
Decibel scale 54–55
Decision making 185–186,
  191
Declarative memory 123
Dehydration 34, 210, 212
Delany, Bessie 183
Delany, Sadie 183
Delirium 226
Delphic oracle 84
Dementia
  causes and types 148–150
  definition 227
  and diet 212
  early stages 140
  exercise for 214
  prevention efforts 37, 150,
    153–155
  role of body fat 207
  social isolation 37
Dementia with Lewy bodies
  (disease) 150
Dendrites 10–12, 22, 152, 227
Depression
  aging 177–179
  and diet 212
  exercise for 32
  neurotransmitter balance
    36–37
  treatment 174
Desimone, Robert 109
Diabetes 34
Diamond, Marian 7–8
Diencephalon 19–20, 227
Diet 204–213
  antioxidants 209
  for better hearing 56
  fish oil 37
  for flexibility 68
  glucose 205, 207
  moderation 213
  nutrients 205
  for optimism 207–208
  for studying and test-taking
    128
  variety 208
  and verbal fluency 96
  whole brain health 37
Digestion 19
Dimoka, Angelika 185–186
Dizziness 78–83
Dopamine 13, 45, 117
Dorsolateral prefrontal cortex
  186
Dreaming 188
Driving 26, 53, 118–119, 223
Drugs 34, 117, 174
Dudukovic, Nicole 128
Duma, Stefan 224
Dyslexia 22

E

Ear
  eardrum 52, 54, 56, 77
  role in balance 74–75, 77, 78
  role in hearing 52, 54
  see also Hearing
Earbuds 55
Easterling, Ray 222
Elderly see Aging
Electroencephalographs (EEGs) 189
Embryo, brain development 21–23
Endocrine system 164, 166
Endorphin 13
Epictetus (Greek philosopher) 195, 196
Epilepsy patients 20, 66
Epinephrine see Adrenaline
Episodic memories 123–124
Ericsson, K. Anders 129, 130–131
Evolving brain
  memory 121–123, 135, 137, 200
  negativity bias 160–162
Executive function 17, 98, 100, 101, 166
Exercise
  aerobic 33, 215
  for balance 79–83
  for brain function 213–216
  dementia prevention 214
  for eyes 45–47, 49, 50
  for flexibility 69, 70–73
  for hearing 58
  living smart 213–216
  for memory 32, 157–159
  for self-esteem 36
  weight-bearing 215
  whole brain health 33
Experience-dependent brain development 9
Experience-expectant brain development 9
Explicit memories 123–124
Eye 44–52
  aging 48, 50–52
  exercises 45–47, 49, 50
  role in balance 74–75
  see also Vision
Eyewitnesses 121, 200

F

Faces, and name memory 137–138
Faces, inability to recognize see Prosopagnosia
Faintness 78
Faloon, Steve 129
Fat 207
Fetus, brain development 22

Fiction reading 178
Fish 37, 212
Fish oil 37, 212
Flanagan, Owen 188
Flashbulb memories 124
Flexibility 68–74
Focus, visual 50
Foer, Joshua 130–131, 137–138, 157
Football 221, 222, 224
Forebrain 227
Franklin, Benjamin 51
Free radicals 209, 227
Free will 30
Freud, Sigmund 188
Frontal lobe 16–17, 21, 145, 194, 227
  see also Prefrontal cortex
Frontotemporal dementia 150
Future brain 225

G

Gage, Phineas 19
Gamma-aminobutyric acid (GABA) 13
Ganglia 227
Garstecki, Dean 55
Genetics 41
Giffords, Gabrielle "Gabby" 95
Gilbert, Daniel 162
Ginkgo biloba 155
Glial cells (neuroglia) 10, 23, 228
Glossary 226–229
Glucose 205, 207
Glutamine 13
Green, Cynthia R. 154
Green, Shawn 115
Gutenberg, Johannes 138

H

Haiku 94
Handford, Martin 109
Hanson, Rick 161, 182
Having Our Say (Delany and Delany) 183
Hearing 52, 54–56, 58
  see also Ear
Hearing loss
  age-related 56, 58, 228
  noise-induced 52, 54–55
Heart-brain connection 33
Heartbeat 21
Helmets 223, 224
Hemispheres 14, 16, 95, 189
Hemorrhagic stroke 149–150, 216, 218
Henner, Marilu 158
Hepler, John 41
Hippocampus
  and blood sugar level 205
  definition 227

  in limbic system 18
  neuron growth 18
  removal 20
  role in memory 20, 124, 142
  and stress 36, 169
HM (Henry Molaison) 20, 124
Hokemeyer, Paul L. 117
Homer Simpson gene 41
Hope, Tony 198
Hubel, David 9
Hugging 168
Hypertension (high blood pressure) 219
Hyperthymesia 158
Hypothalamus 166, 227

I

Illusions 107–109
Imagination 178
Immune system 181–182, 193–194
Implants 83
Implicit memories 123, 124
Information overload 167, 186, 188
Information processing speed 26
Inhibitory function 26
Inner ear 78
Insight (phenomenon) 189, 191
Insula 87–89, 227
Ischemic stroke 149–150, 216, 218
Isolation, social 37, 56, 147

J

Jackson, John Hughlings 66
Jefferson, Thomas 88
Jepson, Stephen 74
Jigsaw puzzles 111
Jiminy Cricket deficiency syndrome 17
Johnson, Samuel 43
Joint health 68
Juggling 76

K

Kakalios, James 23
Kaku, Michio 225
Kalil, Ronald E. 25
Kant, Immanuel 42
Katz, Lawrence 35, 60, 63, 153
Killingsworth, Matthew 162
Krebs, Emil 88

L

Language 84–103
  aging brain 85–87, 96–97
  Brain Boosters 86, 89, 90, 93, 94, 99
  cognitive fitness 38

insula 87–89
learning a second language 40, 98–103
phonological priming 91–92
polyglots 88
tip-of-the-tongue experiences 85–87, 91–92
verbal fluency 92–93, 95–98
Laughter 37
Lazar, Sara 170, 172
Learning
in children 9
increasing neural connections 7–8, 14, 82
life-long 9
strengthening brain organ 7–8, 40
Learning Later, Living Greater (Nordstrom) 181
Left hemisphere 14, 16, 95
Lewis, Carole B. 80–81
Life expectancy 227
Lifelogging 141
Lightheadedness 78
Limbic system 18
Limitless (movie) 23
Linkenauger, Sally A. 108–109
Lion's Breath (yoga exercise) 176
Living smart 204–225
Brain Boosters 206, 211, 215, 217, 219, 223
concussion 218–225
diet 204–213
exercise 213–216
stroke 216–217
Loci, method of 131–133, 135, 137, 228
Locke, John 42
"Locked-in" syndrome 100
London, England, cabdrivers 18
Loneliness 177–178
Long-term memory 26, 123–124, 144
Longevity 227
Lorenz, Edward 28–29
Luria, A. R. 133–135
Lust, Barbara 101

M
Magic Eye stereograms 110, 112
Maguire, Eleanor 18
The Man Who Mistook His Wife for a Hat (Sacks) 105
Mankato, Minnesota nun study 40, 101
Map-reading skills 114
Mar, Raymond 178
Marine Corps, U.S. 56
McCredie, Scott 77
McMahon, Jim 221

Medications
drug abuse 34, 117
for negative mental states 174
Meditation 170–172, 190
Mediterranean diet 208
Medulla oblongata 21, 74, 227
Memory 120–159
aging brain 26, 141–142, 145–150
in Alzheimer's 146–147
Brain Boosters 122, 127, 130, 136, 139, 143, 144, 152, 156
categorization 139
chunking 126, 128–130
contests 137, 157
evolution 121–123, 135, 137, 200
exercise for 32, 157–159
genetics 41
hippocampus 20
limitations 157
long-term 26, 123–124, 144
Magic Number Seven 125–126
Mark Twain's game 125
memorable house tour 132–133
method of loci 131–133, 135, 137, 228
mnemonics 129, 138
and mood 200–203
and music 97–98
name recollection 137–138
number recollection 129–131
optimal health 150–151, 153–155, 157
perfect memory 133–135, 158
plasticity 98, 124, 182
print's impact 138, 140
short-term 123
storage 120–123
stress's impact 36, 169
studying for a test 128
training 151
types of memory 123–124
working 26
Memory palace *see* Method of loci
Meninges 227
Merzenich, Michael 82
Method of loci 131–133, 135, 137, 228
Midbrain 228
Military service
noise-induced hearing loss 54, 56
Miller, George 125–126
Mindfulness 190
Mirror, mirror (perception exercise) 49
Mirror box therapy 112

Mnemonics 129, 138
Moffat, Marilyn 80–81
Molaison, Henry (HM) 20, 124
Monet, Claude 181
Monfils, Marie 203
Mood and creativity 160–183
achieving balance 170–173
adolescence 25
aging 177–179
Alzheimer's 147
Brain Boosters 163, 165, 168, 171, 175, 176, 180
brain chemicals 36–37
creativity 165, 179–183
and diet 207–208
memory links 200–203
negativity bias 160–162
professional help 174–177
see also Stress
Moonwalking With Einstein (Foer) 130–131, 157
Moral behavior 19
Motion circuits 66, 68
Motor cortex 25, 66, 83
Motor neuron 228
Motor skills 68
Movement 64–83
balance 74–75, 77–83
Brain Boosters 67, 69, 73, 76, 79
brain circuitry 66, 68
coordinated by cerebellum 20–21
dizziness 78–83
flexibility 68–74
motion circuits 66, 68
muscle fibers 65
neurons 66, 68
Multivitamins 212
Muscles 65
Music
brain fitness 40
and hearing loss 55
and language 97–98
and memory 97–98
tap a tune (Brain Booster) 67
write a love song (Brain Booster) 180
Music therapy 95
Myelin 10, 202
Myelin sheath 228
Myelination 25, 202
Myopia 44–45, 228

N
Names, remembering 137–138
National Football League (NFL) concussions 221, 222
Native Americans, storytelling 135
Navratilova, Martina 72
Neanderthals 75, 77

Necker, Louis Albert 107
Necker cube 107–108
Negativity
   in daydreams 162
   evolutionary bias 160–162
   and longevity 193
   switching to positivity 182,
      195–198
Neural connections
   aging 38
   as buffer against decline 38
   increase through enrichment
      7–8, 38, 82
   number of 11
   prenatal pruning 22
Neural networks 23, 82
Neurobics 153
Neuroglia (glial cells) 10, 23,
   228
Neuron migration 22
Neurons
   aging brain 26, 38
   Alzheimer's 149
   communication 10–14
   definition 228
   growth 18, 22–23
   inhibitory function 26
   number of 10, 11
   prenatal development 22
   role in movement 66, 68
Neuropeptides 181–182
Neuroplasticity see Plasticity
Neurotransmitters
   adjustment through medica-
      tion 174
   aging brain 179
   definition 12, 228
   and mood 36–37
   role 12, 166
   stress-related 164, 166
Newborns, brain development
   22–23
NFL (National Football League)
   concussions 221, 222
Nicotine 33
Nondeclarative memory 123
Nordstrom, Nancy Merz 181
Norepinephrine 13, 164
Nun study 40, 101
Nutrition see Diet

O
Oatley, Keith 178
Obesity 96, 207
Occipital lobe 18, 105, 110
O'Keeffe, Georgia 181
Olfaction 57, 59
Oligodendrocytes 10
Omega-3 fatty acids 37, 212
Online resources 61, 93
Optical illusions 107–109
Optimism see Positivity

Optogenetics 228
Origami 39
Oxygen, use by brain 142

P
Parasympathetic nervous sys-
   tem 170, 228
Parietal lobe 17, 228
Parkinson's disease 68
Perception 37, 43–44, 49, 106,
   108–109
   see also Senses
Perfect memory 133–135, 158
Peripheral nervous system 228
Perspective 107–108
Perspiration 19
Pert, Candace 181–182
Pessimism see Negativity
PET (positron emission tomog-
   raphy) scans 142, 145
"Phantom limb" phenomenon
   112
Phenomenon (movie) 92, 95
Phonological loop 126
Phonological priming 91–92
Photographic memory 133–135
Physics of the future (Kaku) 225
Pitt, Brad 87, 89
Plaque buildup, in Alzheimer's
   149
Plasticity
   aging brains 8, 26–27
   definition 8
   emotional memories 182
   lifelong 181
   London cabdrivers 18
   memory 124
   musical training and mem-
      ory 98
   young brains 8–9, 25
Plato (Greek philosopher) 138,
   140
Poe's Heart and the Mountain
   Climber (Restak) 167
Poetry 94, 156
Polyglots 88
Pons 21, 74, 228
Posit Science games 119
Positivity
   accentuating 182, 193
   improving cognitive function
      194–195
   and longevity 193
   strengthening immune sys-
      tem 193–194
   switching attitude to 194–198
Positron emission tomography
   (PET) scans 142, 145
Post-traumatic stress disorder
   177
Posterior occipital lobes 105
Poverty, impact on children 169

Prefrontal cortex (PFC) 16–17
   adolescent brain 25
   aging brain 26
   definition 228
   executive function 17, 98,
      166
   free will 30
   information overload 186
   moral behavior 19
   myelination 202
   negativity bias 161–162
Prenatal care 22
Presbycusis see Hearing loss,
   age-related
Presbyopia 48, 50, 51, 228
Price, Jill 158
Printing press 138, 140
Proffitt, Dennis R. 108–109
Proprioception 75, 229
Prosopagnosia 105

Q
Quadriplegics 83

R
Ramachandran, Vilayanur S.
   105, 112
Reading
   benefits 178
   and myopia 45
Reality 42
Receptor, definition 229
Record keeping 140
Red wine 210
Reflexes 21
Relaxation 186, 188–189
   see also Meditation
Remembering see Memory
Repetition 152
Respiration see Breathing
Restak, Richard 167, 177, 179
Resveratrol 34, 210
Reynolds, Jeremy 178
RGS14 (gene) 41
Right hemisphere 14, 16, 189
Robots 83
Rogers, Fred 203
Rose, Kathryn 45
Rosetta stone 88

S
"S" (man with perfect memory)
   133–135
Sacks, Oliver 104–105
Schalk, Gerwin 100
Schliemann, Heinrich 88
School
   memories 144
   test-taking 128, 194–195
Seafood 37
Seau, Junior 221, 222
Seizures 20

Selective attention 112–113, 115, 117–119
Semantic memories 123–124
Senses 42–63
  aging 26, 43–44, 48, 59
  augmenting 60–63
  Brain Boosters 47, 49, 50, 53, 57, 61, 62
  focus 44–45, 172–173
  hearing 52, 54–56, 58
  new sensations 60–63
  perceptions 43–44
  processing 121
  smell 57, 59
  taste 59
  touch 59–60, 62
  vision 44–52
Sensory neuron 229
Serotonin 13, 207–208
Seven, as magic number 125–126
"SF" (memory-study subject) 129–131
Shafto, Meredith 86
Shellfish 37
Short-term memory 123
Simonides of Ceos (legend) 131–132
Skin, touch receptors 59–60
Sleep
  deprivation 34, 95–96
  disturbances in elderly 179
  dreaming 188
Smell, sense of 57, 59
Smoking 33
Snowball effect 196–197
Social engagement 175
Social isolation 37, 56, 147
Somatic nervous system 229
Sound processing 52, 54
Spatial navigation 18
Spoon, Nicole 170
Spinal cord 21, 66, 229
Sports 108–109, 218, 220–225
Squirrel monkeys 82
Steen, Derek 112
Stereographs 110
Stimuli 12, 152, 153
Stress
  benefits 36
  long-term exposure 166–167, 169
  negative aspects 36
  physiological effects 34, 36, 164, 166, 169
  professional therapy 174, 176–177
  reduction techniques 168, 170–173
Stress hormones 164, 166, 169, 226
Stretching 69, 70–72

Stroke
  effects 68, 105, 149–150
  incidence 216
  recovery 222
  risk factors 216, 218, 219
  treatment 218, 222
  warning signs 217
Studying for tests 128
Sugar, restricting intake 209
Sunlight, and myopia 45
Sustain your brain 6–27
  aging brain 26–27
  brain anatomy 14, 15
  Brain Boosters 15, 24, 26–27
  brain development 21–23
  brain lobes and functions 16–18
  brain regions and functions 19–21
  brain system 10–11
  learning as fitness regimen 7–8
  memory 18
  neural communication 12–13
  youthful brain 25
Swallow, Khena 178
Sympathetic nervous system 164, 166, 170, 229
Synapses 229
Synesthesia 134, 229

T
Tai chi 80, 83
Taste, sense of 59
Taub, Edward 222
Teenagers 25, 202
Telepathy 100, 225
The Tell-Tale Brain (Ramachandran) 105
Temporal lobe 17–18, 20, 229
Test-taking 128, 194–195
Thalamus 20, 164, 229
Therapy
  cognitive behavioral therapy 174, 176–177
  cognitive therapy 195–198
  constraint induced movement therapy 222
  mirror box therapy 112
  music therapy 95
  vision therapy 110, 112
Thinking 37
Three-dimensional imaging systems 110
Thurber, James 181
Tip-of-the-tongue experiences 85–87, 91–92
Tongue 63
Touch, sense of 59–60, 62
Townshend, Pete 55
Toxins 34

Train Your Mind, Change Your Brain (Begley) 176–177
Transient myopia 45
Tryptophan 208
Twain, Mark 125
Twitter 100

U
Upright posture 66, 68, 75
USA Memory Championship 137

V
Ventricles 229
Verbal fluency 92–93, 95–96
Vertigo 78
Vestibular system 74–75, 77, 79, 229
Video gaming 115, 168
Vision 44–52
  improving 45–47, 49, 50
  perception 44–45, 107–109
  processing 18, 104–105, 110
  selective attention 113
Vision therapy 110, 112
Visual agnosia 104–105
Visual attention (phenomenon) 115
Visual cortex 18, 107, 109, 121
Visual memories 121
Visual scanning 116
Visualization 172
Vitality 36–37
Vitamin C 68, 208
Vitamin supplements 212

W
Waldo (cartoon figure) 109
Walking 32
Water consumption 210, 212
Weather patterns, modeling 28–29
Weight-bearing exercise 215
Wernicke's aphasia 84–85
Where's Waldo? (Handford) 109
The Who (rock band) 55
Wiesel, Torsten 9
Williams, Justin 100
Wilson, Adam 100
Wine 210
Witnesses, reliability 121, 200
Witt, Jessica K. 108–109
Woods, Tiger 25
Writing, and memory 138, 140

Y
Yoga 73, 176
Youthful brains 8–9, 25
  see also Adolescents; Children

Z
Zacks, Jeffrey 178
Zhang Sanfeng 80

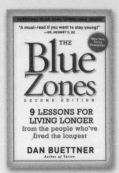
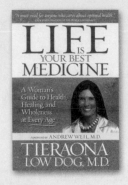
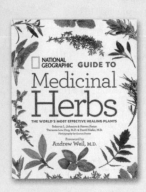
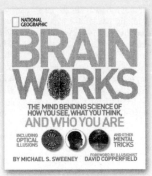

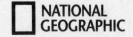